PREVENTION'S
MEDICAL HEALING YEARBOOK
1991

Edited by Mark Bricklin, Editor
and Sharon Stocker, Associate Editor
Prevention® Magazine

Written by the Staff of Rodale Press

Rodale Press, Emmaus, Pennsylvania

The following chapters were adapted from and reprinted by permission of *Medical Self-Care* magazine, P.O. Box 1000, Pt. Reyes, CA 94956: Chapter 10, "A New Weapon against Alcoholism" ("The New Intervention Approach to Alcohol Addiction," January/February 1990); Chapter 22, "How the Stress Experts Deal with Theirs" ("How the Stress Experts Deal with Theirs," January/February 1990); Chapter 18, "The Politics of Home Testing" ("The FDA and Home Medical Tests," November/December 1989); Chapter 24, "Is Your Medication Zapping Your Hair?" ("Common Drugs Cause Hair Loss," November/December 1989); Chapter 38, "Don't Get Skinned" ("Acne and Wrinkle Drug Hazards," September/October 1989); Chapter 25, "Fighting Athlete's Foot" ("Athlete's Foot: The Fungus among Us," September/October 1989); Chapter 30, "Pap Test Update" ("Pap Tests," March/April 1989).

The following chapters were adapted from the *Wall Street Journal*, November 13, 1989. Reprinted by permission of the *Wall Street Journal*, Copyright © 1989 Dow Jones & Company, Inc. All rights reserved worldwide: Chapter 1, "Major Medical Breakthroughs" ("Causes and Cures"); Chapter 4, "Medical Mimics" ("Medical Mimics"); Chapter 19, "The High Costs of High-Tech ("A Two-Edged Sword"); Chapter 20, "Good-Bye to the Bedside Manner" ("Out of Touch"); Chapter 21 "Diagnosis in the Fast Lane" ("Rapid Results").

Chapter 6, "Ironing Out Erratic Heartbeats," was adapted from *Heart Rhythms*, by Jeffrey Rothfeder, copyright© 1989 by Jeffrey Rothfeder. Reprinted by permission of Little, Brown & Co.

Chapter 7, "A Guide to High Blood Pressure Drugs," was adapted from *Lower Your Blood Pressure and Live Longer*, by Marvin Moser, copyright © 1989 by Marvin Moser, M.D., and G. S. Sharpe Communications, Inc. Reprinted by permission of Villard Books, a division of Random House, Inc.

Chapter 16, "Take Charge of Choosing a Surgeon," was adapted from *Taking Charge of Your Medical Care*, by Lawrence C. Horowitz, copyright © 1988 by LCH Enterprises, Inc. Reprinted by permission of Random House, Inc.

If you have any questions or comments concerning this book, please write:
Rodale Press
Book Reader Service
33 East Minor Street
Emmaus, PA 18098

ISBN 0–87857–919–2 hardcover

Distributed in the book trade by St. Martin's Press

2   4   6   8   10   9   7   5   3   1   hardcover

Notice

This book is intended as a reference volume only, not as a medical manual or guide to self-treatment. If you suspect that you have a medical problem, we urge you to seek competent medical help. Keep in mind that nutritional and health needs vary from person to person, depending on age, sex, health status, and total diet. The information here is intended to help you make informed decisions about your health, not as a substitute for any treatment that may have been prescribed by your doctor.

Contributors to
Prevention's Medical Healing Yearbook 1991

WRITERS: Pamela Boyer, Mark L. Fuerst, Steven Lally, Gale Maleskey, Gloria McVeigh, Joe Mullich, Kerry Pechter, Cathy Perlmutter, Porter Shimer, Sharon Stocker

PRODUCTION EDITOR: Jane Sherman

DESIGNER: Glen Burris

BOOK LAYOUT: Lisa Farkas

COVER DESIGN: Lisa Farkas

COPY EDITOR: Candace Levy

ASSOCIATE RESEARCH CHIEF, *PREVENTION* MAGAZINE: Pamela Boyer

OFFICE MANAGER: Roberta Mulliner

OFFICE PERSONNEL: Barbara Bach, Karen Earl-Braymer

Contents

Part I
Frontiers in Medical Research

An explosion in basic science research is yielding
mind-boggling diagnostic and treatment tools: radioactive tracers that seek out and target cancer cells, ultraviolet light that destroys enemy cells believed to cause
multiple sclerosis, and much more.

The concept of an effective natural cancer treatment
with no pain and minimal expense is seductive. We're
not quite there yet, but scientists are reaching for the
goal with vitamins A, B, C, D, and E against a variety
of malignancies.

An update on the latest ways to help your body heal
itself as quickly as possible, from home-care tips to
nip colds, cure insomnia, and speed wound healing to
medical techniques for bouncing back after surgery,
patching hernias, and more.

Part II
Advances in Heart Health

Part III
Top Disease-Fighting Strategies

Ten years ago your only choices were to let stones pass through on their own or to undergo major surgery. Thank goodness modern medical advances in prevention and treatment offer a less painful alternative.

Part IV
Finding the Best Medical Treatment

With so many options, trying to locate a clinic that can best serve your needs can be maddening. Those who need top-notch arthritis treatment will appreciate this list of the country's best clinics.

Most of us aren't used to questioning authority—especially when it comes from an M.D. But learning to ask questions firmly and diplomatically beforehand can make the difference between life and death for you once you're on the operating table.

Where do you go when you've been examined by every type of specialist in the book, been given a plethora of medical tests, and spent hundreds of dollars and hours pursuing an answer, but find your problem defies explanation? To one of the nation's top-notch, multispecialty "superclinics," of course.

The technology for home tests for strep throat, urinary tract and vaginal infections, cholesterol levels, and others is already available, but the FDA and many medical authorities don't believe the public is capable of using them responsibly.

Part V
The Perils of Technology

The Blue Cross and Blue Shield Association estimates
that between $6 billion and $18 billion a year is wasted
on unnecessary medical tests. Expensive machines, it
seems, must be kept in constant use to justify their
initial cost.

A 1940s doctor laments the loss of medical training
that served to extend the physician's own senses—a
honing of observational skills that made bedside diagnosis warm and personal.

Primary-care physicians can now perform many sophisticated medical tests in their office. While that can
spell quicker results for patients, excessive numbers of
unnecessary tests suggest that at least some doctors
are using the tests to pad their wallets.

Part VI
Updates on Everyday Health Care

By now everyone's pretty much accepted that stress is
impossible to avoid entirely. Even so, many of us have
yet to develop our own personal coping strategies.
Here you'll find some hints from the experts.

Chapter 23
Vision Quests... 204
Experts from the American Academy of Ophthalmol-
ogy highlight the latest breakthroughs for treating
middle-age eye problems like glaucoma, presbyopia,
cataracts, detached retinas, and macular degeneration.

Chapter 24
Is Your Medication Zapping Your Hair?................. 214
Few pharmaceutical companies broadcast that many
prescription drugs may cause hair to thin. Nevertheless, it's true. Check this partial list of culprits for your
medication. If it's not here, double-check with your
doctor just to be sure.

Chapter 25
Fighting Athlete's Foot...................................... 217
Athletes aren't the only ones who pick up this nasty,
itchy, persistent fungus infection. Here's a how-to
guide for anyone who wishes to identify and exorcise
the annoying condition pronto.

Chapter 26
Cure Chronic Hyperventilation........................... 220
It may not be a heart attack, but it sure feels like one.
And without proper diagnosis, the chronic hyperven-
tilator can spend years going from doctor to doctor
seeking help. Here are steps to stop the vicious circle.

Chapter 27
Is Your Iron High or Low?.................................. 226
Taking iron supplements when they aren't needed can
lead to an overload called hemosiderosis—with symptoms like skin bronzing, diabetes, enlarged heart,
heart arrhythmias, loss of libido, abdominal pain, and
arthritis.

Part VII
Women's Health Newsfront

Part VIII
Beauty Therapies for the 1990s

Chapter 32
Spot-Reduction Weight Loss: At Last 267
Liposuction can mean quick, easy, and effective
weight loss for the right person with the right surgeon. These guidelines will help you decide whether
or not you're a good candidate and, if so, how to find
"doctor right."

Chapter 33
Fuzz Busters.. 274
Prevention magazine's beauty editor gives a personal
report on her experience with electrolysis, sharing
with you what to expect from the procedure and how
you can avoid common pitfalls.

Chapter 34
Don't Get Skinned 279
Anyone thinking of trying out the new vitamin A
drugs that fight acne and wrinkles should read up
first. Some of the side effects can be dangerous, especially for women.

INTRODUCTION

Medical Care Options: Don't Let the Numbers Get You Down

Lots of people would just as soon not know the details of their illness—what's being tested, what's being diagnosed, what's being prescribed. Perhaps they're afraid that knowing too much will only reveal the worst, so they take refuge in the small comfort gained by ignoring the fact that whatever it is just might be serious.

Others are afraid to speak up and ask questions that demand even brief explanations. One patient declined to tell her referred doctor what other medications she was on when he asked because she was "afraid to waste his time." An extreme case, it's true, but most of us can identify with the sentiment behind the woman's concern. We know and respect that doctors are busy people, so we hesitate to take more of their time than absolutely necessary.

Perhaps the most common reason, however, is how overwhelming—even agonizing—we find the vast array of treatment options these days. Take just one important example, heart health. It used to be that if you had heart trouble like angina, you took nitroglycerin. Now, cardiologists and heart surgeons experiment with and implement innumerable sophisticated techniques that help control, even reverse, coronary blockage: the "excimer" laser; balloon angioplasty; Roto-Rooter devices; bypass surgery; drugs like beta-blockers, cholestyramine, and niacin; exercise; diet (including oat bran, fish oil, and a superlow fat intake); aspirin; and stress-reduction techniques like meditation and guided imagery.

No question about it—the explosion of technological discoveries, not only in heart health but in numerous major diseases, is incredibly exciting. But when it comes to which technique or combination is best for your particular situation, opinions among the experts can vary considerably. Medical care choices are simply not as black and white as they used to be, making it increasingly important for us as patients to participate when critical decisions are being made.

And that's what *Prevention's Medical Healing Yearbook* for 1991 is all about. Chapter after chapter describes the latest and most exciting lifesaving procedures, to provide you with the facts that help in making decisions. The pros and cons of various techniques, laid out clearly, simply, and practically, help you weigh the evidence for yourself— because it's *your* health that's in the balance.

Sharon Stocker
Associate Editor
Prevention Magazine

CHAPTER 1

Major
Medical
Breakthroughs

A new understanding of how the body works is yielding lifesaving techniques for a host of major diseases.

Those over age 35 might remember the day in August 1963 when the nation was saddened by the death of President John F. Kennedy's infant son. The child, born 5½ weeks prematurely, died of severe respiratory distress less than two days after birth; as often happens in premature births, the infant's lungs hadn't yet developed the lubricant-like film that coats the air sacs and prevents them from collapsing.

Today, he might have lived.

A quarter of a century after the president's son died, medical researchers are finally coming up with a way to prevent such tragic deaths, which occur at the rate of

5,000 a year. As many as six different versions of synthetic coatings for infants' lungs are just now emerging from research laboratories.

That may not seem all that surprising; new medical treatments are announced almost daily. But the simultaneous development of six medications is more than just another medical advancement. It is also a dramatic illustration of how medical technology has changed over the last few years—and how it will leave its mark in the 1990s.

Until recently, medical research was largely a matter of discovery by trial and error. By contrast, the medical technology welling up out of today's laboratories is grounded in a new understanding of how the human body works and why it goes wrong.

Basic discoveries in how the body controls the growth of cells, for instance, are opening a variety of treatments for cancer, the healing of wounds, and the control of blood disorders. Unraveling the complexities of the human immune system is leading to advances against not only cancer but also arthritis, multiple sclerosis, diabetes, AIDS, and innumerable lesser-known disorders. And basic breakthroughs into the mysteries of the genes are about to change the treatment of heart disease dramatically and may soon lead to cures or prevention of muscular dystrophy, cystic fibrosis, Alzheimer's disease, alcoholism, and perhaps scores of other ailments that have defied medical science.

Even the hardware of medicine is being built increasingly on foundations of basic biological and physiological knowledge. The new magnetic resonance imaging (MRI) scanners that deliver spectacularly detailed pictures of the interior of the human body are based on new knowledge of how atoms in living tissue behave under the influence of magnetic fields. Lasers are being brought to bear on problems ranging from nearsightedness to heart attacks because of new understandings of how living tissue reacts to the powerful light beams.

Here is a brief look at how this explosion in basic knowledge is changing the diagnosis and treatment of some of the major diseases.

Arthritis and Other Inflammatory Diseases

New knowledge of what causes inflammation of tissues is opening potential new therapies for rheumatoid arthritis and other inflammatory disorders.

A new class of drugs appears to prevent the tissues from making the substances (called leukotrienes) that cause inflammation. These new drugs work differently from cortisone, aspirin, and the nonsteroidal anti-inflammatory drugs like ibuprofen (Motrin) that are the current mainstays of treating inflammatory disorders.

Several leukotriene blockers are being tested against arthritis, psoriasis, and inflammatory bowel disorders like Crohn's disease and ulcerative colitis. An initial, short-term test with one experimental leukotriene blocker, made by Pfizer, Inc., produced favorable changes in body chemistry of 800 rheumatoid arthritis patients.

Sufferers of the inflammatory bowel disorders also may soon benefit from an old drug. Methotrexate, a 40-year-old anticancer drug now being used for arthritis, produced improvements in 16 of 21 patients with either Crohn's disease or ulcerative colitis in an early test in Seattle.

In the future, there's the chance that a monoclonal antibody, similar to those developed for cancer, might be wielded against inflammatory diseases. Biotechnology companies are developing monoclonal antibodies that would knock out the white blood cells that are mistakenly attacking and inflaming the body's own tissues. Such an autoimmune attack on the collagen of the joints is believed to cause the inflammation of rheumatoid arthritis.

Cancer

The problem of detecting hidden patches of cancer cells is about to be solved by monoclonal antibodies. "Monoclonals" are man-made versions of the antibodies the human immune system launches against any foreign protein, such as a virus, that endangers the body. A monoclonal antibody can be designed that attaches itself only to one specific type of cancer cell and no other cell, normal or cancerous.

Biotechnology companies have developed and are mass-producing a dozen different monoclonal antibodies. Several selectively seek out only colon cancer cells while others are specific to ovarian, breast, lung, or prostate cancers.

For cancer detection, the companies have learned how to glue radioactive tracers to the monoclonals. Radiation detectors can reveal where the tagged monoclonals go in the body, thus revealing the location of patches of cancer cells too small to be seen by x-rays or MRI scans. Used before surgery, the monoclonals can guide the surgeon to hidden deposits of cancer cells that might otherwise be missed. After surgery or chemotherapy, they can reveal whether a second operation or round of chemotherapy is necessary, often obviating the need for exploratory surgery.

At the same time, a score of therapeutic monoclonals, each of which selectively attacks and destroys a particular type of cancer, either are in clinical trial or are about to begin such human testing.

Cancer patients also will benefit from the discovery of substances the body normally produces to trigger the multiplication of particular cells. "Colony stimulating factors" (CSFs), for example, stimulate the multiplication of colonies of bone marrow cells. Destruction of the bone marrow is what limits the use of powerful anticancer drugs to less than curative doses. Cancer researchers now believe that the CSFs, by speeding the recovery of the bone marrow, will allow the use of higher, more effective doses of the anticancer chemicals.

Other cell stimulators, called interleukins, are being used to activate white blood cells that normally attack cancers but that seem to be sluggish or quiescent in cancer patients. One widely publicized "killer cell" activator, interleukin-2, has produced remissions in a small percentage of advanced cancer patients who failed to respond to any other therapy.

Heart Disease

The newfound ability to locate and identify genes is uncovering an astonishingly large number and variety of inherited genetic defects that render people susceptible to heart attacks. The score, or more, of defects found so far all seem to alter, in one way or another, the body's normal processing of fats and cholesterol. The aberrations lead to a buildup of the cholesterol-rich deposits in the coronary arteries that, in turn, eventually leads to a heart attack.

Scientists are trying to discover how widespread each defect is in the population. They hope to introduce new blood tests that could tell whether an individual has inherited a genetic susceptibility to coronary heart disease. The genetic blood tests ultimately may replace the present cholesterol blood test that misses many people with a genetic predisposition to coronary heart disease because their total blood cholesterol level appears normal. Genetic tests would allow heart specialists to tailor their diet and drug prescriptions to the individual rather than spend months in trying each therapy to see which, if any, works best in each patient.

Heart surgeons are developing new "Roto-Rooters" to clear out coronary arteries already clogged with deposits. At present, such heart patients have either coronary bypass surgery or balloon angioplasty, in which inflating a tiny balloon in the artery squeezes open a passage for blood flow. A new device, using a rotating, cylinder-shaped blade, shaves the deposits away; it's being tested to see whether it's better than the balloon idea.

Trials are under way to see whether the new "excimer" laser can etch the deposits away with its invisible beam. The excimer laser is so delicate it can etch designs on a butterfly's wings; it should avoid the danger that hampers other lasers in artery unclogging—that of accidentally burning a hole in the artery.

Infant
Respiratory Distress

The prevention of collapsing lungs in premature babies is advancing rapidly. Burroughs Wellcome Co. has distributed a sterile, man-made powder to hospitals around the country. When reconstituted with sterile water at the cribside, the powder produces a white, foamy liquid. Administered through a ventilator tube to the lungs of a premature infant in respiratory distress, the foamy liquid forms the soapy film that is missing from the tiny lungs. Tests on more than 2,000 premature infants show that the synthetic surfactant, as it's called, cut the number of deaths from respiratory distress by a third.

Meanwhile, two other lung surfactants, one being developed by Abbott Laboratories and another by ONY, Inc., a small, university-based company in Buffalo, are nearing the market. And, according to *Physicians' Weekly*, a news publication for doctors, at least three other synthetic surfactants are in the development stage.

Multiple Sclerosis

The progressive crippling of multiple sclerosis (MS) is the result of the immune system's steadily—and mistakenly—destroying the outer covering of the nerves. High doses of radiation that dampen the immune system appear to retard the progress of the disease in some patients treated at a Newark, New Jersey, center.

A half-dozen medical centers have begun testing the idea of treating MS by separating the watery part of the blood—the plasma—and replacing it with plasma substitutes. This temporarily gets rid of the antibodies and other toxic immune elements that attack the nerves. Initial results indicate this plasma exchange, combined with immune-suppression drugs, can mitigate the relapse of the disease that periodically afflicts certain MS patients.

A similar but more exotic idea is being tried at the University of Pennsylvania. It is believed that malfunctioning of the white blood cells known as T-cells is why the nerves are being attacked in MS. So in the experiment, MS patients are given a drug that makes the T-cells sensitive to ultraviolet light. A pint of blood is removed, and the part containing the T-cells is exposed to ultraviolet light. The T-cells are so changed by the light that when they are returned to the body, the immune system regards them as "foreign" cells and destroys them. It's a way to selectively knock out the troublesome T-cells without dampening the entire immune system as drugs and radiation do.

Prenatal Diagnosis

Earlier and quicker diagnosis of defects in the fetus are in the offing for pregnant women. The new chorionic villus sampling (CVS), in which cells are obtained from the developing placenta, is proving easier and almost as good in detecting defective fetuses as amniocentesis, which uses amniotic fluid. The simpler CVS procedure can be performed at 7 to 10 weeks of pregnancy— instead of 16 to 18 weeks for amniocentesis—when abortion, if chosen, is easier.

Added to the CVS advance is another called polymerase chain reaction (PCR) that can help provide a diagnosis of a genetic disorder such as cystic fibrosis or muscular dystrophy within a couple of hours instead of two weeks. The PCR is a technique for taking DNA from only a few fetal cells and rapidly copying it until there is enough to detect a defective gene. It also can be used to tell a woman, on a "diagnosis-while-you-wait" basis, whether she is a carrier of an inherited disease.

Enlarged Prostate

Urologists are testing nonsurgical treatments for aging males' most common health problem: an enlarged prostate gland that interferes with urination. The usual treatment for this problem is a 20-minute operation in which a catheter is used to surgically reopen a channel for the urethra.

Now some urologists and radiologists are borrowing an idea from heart surgeons: They use a catheter to insert a tiny balloon through the urethra into the enlarged prostate. The balloon is inflated for several minutes, reopening the channel. Advocates say the procedure is easier and cheaper than conventional surgery.

Another experiment involves temporarily inserting a tiny microwave probe through the urethra into the prostate. The microwaves heat the prostate. In one test, hour-long treatments semiweekly seemed to improve 20 of 21 men.

At least two drugs are being tested to see whether they can reduce the size of enlarged prostates without surgery.

One drug, from Merck & Co., blocks the formation of testosterone, the male sex hormone that causes prostate enlargement. An enzyme inhibitor from Abbott Laboratories also is showing some promise in reducing prostate size in early tests.

Surgery

The discovery of a multitude of "growth factors" used by the human body is leading to faster healing of surgical incisions. Several of the tissue growth factors are being produced in quantity by genetic engineering. One such factor—applied to skin wounds where small patches had been removed for grafting to other parts of the body— caused the wounds to heal 20 percent faster than untreated wounds nearby.

Scarless wound healing after surgery—a kind of Holy Grail of plastic surgery—may someday be possible. Surgeons who have been operating on fetuses to correct anatomical defects before birth have noticed there aren't any scars on the child at birth. Researchers are now trying to find out how fetal wound healing differs from "normal" wound healing.

Transplants

The problem of obtaining human livers for transplanting to dying patients, particularly children, is being eased. Patients dying of liver diseases have had to wait for a donor to die before a transplantable liver could be obtained. This has been a major problem for children who have to wait until another child dies to obtain a liver small enough to be transplanted.

The liver, however, is a regenerating organ, and it can be divided into several pieces, each of which will regenerate into a full-size, functioning liver. So surgeons are beginning to use each liver from a dead donor for transplants to two patients. Moreover, the half or quarter of an adult liver is small enough to be placed in a child, where it will function and grow with the child. It also makes it possible for a living parent to donate a segment of his or her liver for transplanting to a small son or daughter.

Meanwhile, a new chemical solution developed at the University of Wisconsin is increasing the length of time that livers can be preserved outside the body to 11 to 12 hours from 4 to 5 hours, thereby increasing the chances of getting a dead donor's organ to a needy recipient.

CHAPTER 2

Vitamins against Cancer

Nutrition can be used for more than prevention, researchers are finding.

Hydroxyurea. Mercaptopurine. Cyclophosphamide. One thing all cancer drugs seem to have in common is their hard-to-spell names.

Or do they? How about A? D? E? These aren't fancy new drugs—they're plain old vitamins. Yet when administered by scientists in large doses, some vitamins may act like drugs, or work with standard cancer-fighting drugs. It isn't clear yet whether the research into this futuristic notion of vitamin chemotherapy will ever pan out. But if the research is successful, chemotherapy could be much easier to take—and a lot easier to spell.

Here's the latest on what scientists have learned so far.

Retinoids against Skin Cancer

Several synthetic forms of vitamin A, collectively called retinoids, have been tested as treatments for skin cancer. They've mostly been pitted against the two skin cancers known as basal-cell and squamous-cell carcinoma. In several tests—just in the experimental stage—oral doses of retinoids have been effective against these carcinomas because retinoids accumulate primarily in the skin.

Most of the studies performed so far have been small, but the results are encouraging. These skin cancers, like all the others that retinoids have been used against, are unlikely to regress on their own. So researchers think that even though their tests are preliminary and have no control groups, the retinoids are probably responsible for the positive effects.

The retinoids etretinate (*eh-TRET-tin-ate*) and isotretinoin (*EYE-so-tret-in-OH-in*) have been used to treat basal-cell carcinoma. In three separate studies on a total of 56 people, 23 showed a partial regression of cancer (the tumors shrank), and five showed complete regression (disappeared). This is an overall response rate of 50 percent, meaning that half the people experienced some decrease in the number or size of tumors.

Once treatment was completed, though, many of the cancers returned. This suggests that regular doses of retinoids may be required for a "cure." Among other things, doctors are conducting studies to determine the best maintenance dose: one that minimizes drying of skin and mucous-membranes, the main side effect.

Researchers are having better luck using oral retinoids against squamous-cell carcinoma. In four small studies, a total of 14 squamous-cell patients were treated with etretinate (4 patients), isotretinoin (9 patients), or arotinoid (1 patient). Six of the 14 had partial remission (tumors reduced in size) or temporary remission (tumors shrank or stopped growing for a short time); another 4 had complete, sustained remissions of the squamous-cell tumors. That adds up to a 71 percent response from an admittedly small sample.

Both basal-cell and squamous-cell carcinomas are relatively easy to cure with surgical removal (used in 90 percent of cases), radiation therapy, or tissue destruction with extreme heat or cold. So why all this fuss about retinoids?

Surgery and other tissue-destroying therapies leave scars. That's not a big problem for a person with one tumor on the back of a hand. But a majority of people with carcinoma have several tumors on areas of the body that are regularly exposed to the tumor-inducing ultraviolet rays of the sun: not only the hands, but the head and neck as well.

Retinoids don't leave scars: Tumors shrink away and normal tissue fills in. That's especially valuable in advanced disease. "One patient had severe, disfiguring tumors on his neck and nose. After six months on isotretinoin, the neck tumor had shrunk to a small, flat lesion. And the nose tumor had shrunk by 70 percent, with preliminary rebuilding of his all-but-eroded nose," explains Scott M. Lippman, M.D., of the Hematology/Oncology Department of M. D. Anderson Cancer Center at the University of Texas, in Houston.

Retinoids have also been tested against malignant melanoma, a more serious form of skin cancer. Preliminary results from a small study of 20 people with advanced melanoma showed some shrinkage of tumors in 3 people. It's far from a cure, but it's a glimmer of hope against a type of cancer that has been resistant to drugs.

A rare skin cancer called mycosis fungoides (*my-KOH-sis fung-GOY-dees*) has shown good response to retinoid therapy. In five preliminary studies, a total of 78 people with the disease were put on oral isotretinoin. More than half showed at least a partial response. The National Cancer Institute is currently sponsoring a clinical study of isotretinoin in combination with other substances against this cancer.

Battling in the Bloodstream

Synthetic versions of vitamins A and D seem to hold promise in the treatment of myeloid leukemia, a cancer of the white blood cells. Both are currently being tested in preliminary trials.

The main problem in leukemia is that immature white blood cells proliferate in the bloodstream, crowding out normal red and white cells. This causes severe anemia and compromises the immune system. But through a hormonal interaction, vitamins A and D seem to make the immature cells grow up. Mature cells appear to stop their rapid reproduction and are able to carry out their immune-system functions.

Initially the active form of vitamin D was tested, but in high doses this has the unfortunate side effect of causing the body to retain calcium. That could cause complications, including hardening of the vital organs and death. But the synthetic version of vitamin D has a more powerful maturing influence on leukemic cells—and a much-lowered calcium-loading mechanism. In studies on leukemic lab mice, this synthetic compound achieved much better results than pure vitamin D. "Some of the mice treated with synthetic D may actually be cured of their leukemia," reports H. Phillip Koeffler, M.D., professor of medicine at UCLA and one of the leading researchers in this field. However promising that may sound, further studies need to be done before this compound is tested in humans.

Synthetic vitamin A has been tested in humans against leukemia, but not on a widespread scale in this country. A few years ago, American researchers at several centers were involved in a double-blind, randomized trial of 13-*cis* retinoic acid (a retinoid compound) in patients with a pre-leukemic condition called myelodysplastic (*MY-low-dis-PLAS-tik*) syndrome. Problems with the study—including many patients quitting the trial—cast suspicion on the results, according to Dr. Koeffler.

One of the researchers, however, continued the study on his own after the trial ended, and found a significant response. Was the original trial too short? It's hard to say without attempts to duplicate those results. The study also showed physicians that the side effects of retinoid therapy drying can be reduced with doses of vitamin E. More reports have come from abroad. Researchers in China and France have reportedly achieved promising results using *trans*retinoic acid against acute promyelocytic leukemia (APL). Up to 75 percent of patients in Chinese studies went into remission. A French researcher has reportedly duplicated their results.

Other research shows that of seven APL patients (from four different studies) treated with isotretinoin, four had what a review article termed "remarkable responses."

Clearly, there's enough evidence to warrant further research on both synthetic A and D.

Fighting with Folate

Leucovorin (*loo-koh-VOR-rin*) is a synthetic form of the B vitamin folate. It's being used in combination with a cancer drug called fluorouracil (*floor-oh-YOOR-a-sill*), commonly referred to as 5-FU. Currently, 5-FU/leucovorin is in clinical trials against several types of cancer. Researchers hope that someday it may become a standard therapy.

By itself, 5-FU has been used against colon cancer for more than 30 years. It interferes with cancer growth by binding to an enzyme needed for cell reproduction. (Some cancer cells reproduce much faster than normal cells. That's how some tumors grow in relation to surrounding tissue.) But 5-FU alone is only moderately effective.

Leucovorin, though, seems to strengthen the bond between 5-FU and the enzyme. The drug/vitamin combination holds onto the enzyme for a longer period than the drug alone. Fewer free enzymes mean slowed or stopped tumor growth.

5-FU/leucovorin has passed a series of clinical trials to determine its effectiveness against advanced, inoperable colon cancer. In five out of seven studies, 5-FU/leucovorin resulted in tumor shrinkage in two to three times as many patients as 5-FU. In two studies patients lived three to five months longer than patients on the standard treatment.

That may not seem like a giant leap forward, but it paves the way for studies in people with earlier (and more treatable) stages of colon cancer. "That's where we hope to have a real impact on the survival rates," says Susan G. Arbuck, M.D., a research clinician at Roswell Park Memorial Institute, in Buffalo, New York. Dr. Arbuck encourages patients who have surgery for colon cancer (and are at high risk for recurrence) to participate in the National Cancer Institute high-priority clinical trials for colon and rectal cancer.

5-FU/leucovorin is being tested against a variety of other malignancies, including cancers of the stomach, breast, pancreas, head, and neck. To find out more about any of these clinical trials (including your eligibility if you've been diagnosed with cancer), call the National Cancer Institute hotline: (800) 4–CANCER.

Colorectal Protectors?

Colorectal polyps are easy to remove but may recur. That prompted researchers at the Ludwig Institute for Cancer Research, in Toronto, to test the effect of vitamins C and E on polyp recurrence.

Two hundred people who were free of polyps after surgery were split into two groups. One group was given daily supplements of 400 milligrams of vitamin C and 400 milligrams of vitamin E. The other got blank look-alikes (placebos).

After about two years, all the patients were checked for polyp recurrence. The researchers noted a slight reduction in polyp recurrence among the patients receiving vitamins C and E. They stressed that further studies should be performed to rule out the possibility that this was a chance finding.

A further study is under way at six research centers in the United States. About 865 people are enrolled in the trial. The patients are split into four groups: The first gets supplements of vitamins C and E; the second group gets beta-carotene (the plant substance our bodies turn into vitamin A); the third gets C, E, and beta-carotene; and the fourth group gets none of the above. Results from this trial are not expected for several years.

Vitamin A for Oral Health

Some time ago, a report from the British Columbia Cancer Research Center, in Vancouver, announced that vitamin A could heal oral leukoplakias (precancerous sores inside the mouth). The study involved 21 people who chew a tobacco-and-betel-nut mixture known to cause an abundance of leukoplakias. After six months of taking vitamin A supplements, 57 percent of the people showed no detectable disease. And none of the tobacco-betel chewers developed new sores while on the vitamin A. Experts estimate that normally only 5 percent of such sores disappear on their own.

Now word comes from the University of California (Irvine) Clinical Cancer Center and the University of Arizona Cancer Center that a milder form of vitamin therapy has the same effect. Seventeen people with oral leukoplakias were given beta-carotene. Each person took 30 milligrams of supplemental beta-carotene per day for three months. Those whose leukoplakias responded to the treatment were kept on it for an additional three months.

At the end of the study, 2 patients had complete remission of their leukoplakias, and 12 others had partial remissions. Of the remaining 3, one showed no change and the other 2 got worse. Overall, that's an 82 percent positive response rate.

The exciting aspect of this study is that beta-carotene, the safest source of vitamin A, was so effective. Pure vitamin A is toxic in high doses, and even the retinoids have unpleasant side effects (primarily skin problems). But beta-carotene is virtually problem-free, even in high doses. That's because the body converts only as much beta-carotene into vitamin A as is needed at the moment. The excess is harmlessly excreted.

What the Good News Means

Vitamin chemotherapy is a seductive idea: The ultimate goal is an effective natural cancer treatment with no pain and minimal expense. But it's not quite that simple—yet.

Scientists are working steadily to see if any of these treatments will turn out to be effective. And even for the vitamins showing the greatest potential, questions of dosage and side effects must be resolved.

Note, too, that several of the vitamin therapies don't use pure vitamins. Leucovorin and isotretinoin are synthetic chemical equivalents of folate and vitamin A, respectively. Slight alterations in their chemistry make them more efficient treatments and/or reduce dangerous side effects seen in high doses of the original vitamin. These synthetic vitamins are different enough to be treated as drugs by the

Food and Drug Administration. They're available by prescription only.

Until scientists nail down the facts, the best course is to go with what we know. Opt for the proven medical treatments. Have suspected cancer checked by a physician. And try a good defense: There's good scientific evidence that a healthy diet can help prevent the start of certain types of cancer. To use this evidence to your fullest advantage, eat a well balanced, nutrient-dense diet that is low in fat. This includes low-fat meats and poultry, fish, whole-grain products, and generous amounts of fresh fruits and vegetables. If you're on a restricted diet—or need added assurance that you're getting the Recommended Dietary Allowance for vitamins and minerals—you may want to consider taking a multiple supplement.

CHAPTER 3
50-Plus
Fast Relief Remedies

From minor cuts and scrapes to major surgical recovery, these up-to-the-minute tips will help shorten healing time.

These days, time is of the essence: fast food . . . speedy service . . . instant communications. Too much of this rush, rush, rush in everyday life can take its toll on your health. But haste doesn't always make waste. If you're sick or hurt, there's nothing better than a fast-paced remedy that puts healing in high gear.

So here's a comprehensive collection of high-speed healers, some of which are self-care remedies, and others—treatments that medical professionals must help you with.

And all are accessible right now (though some are so

new that their availability is limited). So what are you waiting for? Read on!

To Recover from Back Injuries . . .

These relief methods should give hope to people suffering from certain types of back pain.

Consider microdiskectomy, an alternative to standard disk surgery. It's a way to remove herniated spinal disks by way of a needle-thin probe that both cuts and vacuums away ruptured disk material. It requires an incision only about an inch in length, compared to the approximately 4-inch cut required by standard surgery. It boasts a higher success rate, and it speeds recovery by substantial margins.

One study, which compared 270 microdiskectomies with 270 standard disk surgeries (laminectomies), found that microdiskectomy patients were able to leave the hospital sooner (in an average of 3.7 days compared to 7.1), were able to return to work sooner (in 10.6 weeks compared to 13.4), and enjoyed a success rate of 98 percent compared to 95 percent for the standard open surgery method.

Microdiskectomy is not without its critics, however. Some argue that it is suitable only for patients whose disk herniations remain contained, meaning they have not broken through the disk's outer shell. The procedure also has been criticized for not allowing an adequate view for surgical work to be done. Proponents of the technique disagree, however, saying that surgical vision is superior thanks to the aid of microscopes, and that if further surgery is required, it can be performed subsequent to microdiskectomy in the standard fashion.

All things considered, microdiskectomy is well worth looking into for anyone suffering from the back and leg pain characteristic of spinal-disk herniation. Some patients find they can walk on the same day as the operation, which usually takes only about 30 minutes and requires not stitches but merely a bandage.

Ask your doctor about cutting short the bed rest. Two days of bed rest may be better for recovery than seven. That was the conclusion reached in a study of 203 low-back pain sufferers reported in the *New England Journal of Medicine*. Patients who stayed in bed for only two days missed 45 percent fewer days of work during the following three months than patients who were confined to bed for a full week. All patients suffered from back pain of similar severity, and all had been advised to follow similar instructions on weight loss, the avoidance of heavy lifting and the use of heat for pain relief. Why had less been more? Possibly because more than a few days of bed rest begins to decondition the body in ways that become counterproductive to recovery. (Back pain due to disk herniation or nerve compression may be an exception, the researchers acknowledged.) Most back pain involves only the muscles or ligaments of the back, however, which appear to respond better to motion than rest once the initial pain of injury has subsided.

Try a new "electrical" technique. It can help heal back muscles so people can begin a conditioning program sooner, say researchers from the Hospital for Joint Diseases Orthopedic Institute in New York City. There, a study of 114 people with various back injuries showed that electrical stimulation of the back muscles increased strength and endurance as much as isometric exercise.

It works much like transcutaneous electrical nerve stimulation (TENS) used for pain relief, but with a less potent electrical signal. Pads are placed on the muscles at each side of the lower spine, and the muscles are electrically stimulated so they'll contract and relax in sequence. The action is similar to that produced by isometric exercise, in which muscles are contracted but the body does not move. The treatment helps you get back to your regular workout and normal life quicker than the bed rest that's usually prescribed. Talk to your physicians about availability.

To Heal Burns . . .

From minor burns to serious trauma, this new technology increases the chances of successful healing.

Welcome the option of laboratory-cloned skin. It's the latest lifesaver for patients burned over a large area of their bodies. Regular skin grafting is slow. "Skin regenerates about every 10 to 15 days, so you can't take a graft from an area any sooner than that," says Phil Walters, director of the skin bank at Shriners Burns Institute in Boston.

But cloning the skin can speed things up quite a bit. A relatively small section of unburned tissue can be cloned in a special culture medium to make an unlimited quantity of new skin—50 or even 100 times the surface area of the original! The average cloning period is about 18 to 20 days. When the cloned skin is grafted on, it "takes" with no risk of rejection because it's essentially going back to its source.

Get nourishment from a special nutrient formula. Serious burn patients heal better and faster when given a special formula (either by tube or by mouth) originally concocted at the Shriners Burns Institute in Cincinnati. Most formulas now in use are too high in the wrong kinds of fat and too low in protein, according to registered dietitian Michele M. Gottschlich, Ph.D., one of the formula's inventors. The Shriners' formula is high in protein; zinc; and vitamins A, C, and E. It's also enriched with omega–3 fatty acids (found in fish oil), but it's low in other types of fat.

The Shriners' formula, now commonly available, has been tested against two commonly used formulas. The results of one small trial indicated that the Shriners' formula significantly reduced the length of time severely burned patients stayed in the hospital. It also greatly decreased the incidence of infection.

Chill out the heat. The fastest way to ensure quick healing of minor (first- or second-degree) burns is to cool down the burned area as soon as possible. The best way to do that: Run cold water over the burn. Cooling the burned area limits the damage caused by heat, leading to a shorter recovery time. This method should be used only on burns in which the skin and/or blisters are unbroken. If the skin is broken, use ice encased in a plastic bag. Serious burns, of course, need a doctor's attention.

Gladly accept artificial skin. In very serious burn cases, cloning (which replaces only the outer layer of skin or epidermis) may not be sufficient. To speed healing of deeper layers of skin, the use of artificial skin can't be beat.

The best type of artificial skin was developed by Ioannis

Yannas, Ph.D., professor of polymer science and engineering at the Massachusetts Institute of Technology, and John Burke, M.D., professor of surgery at Harvard Medical School. It includes an outer layer, an artificial epidermis, to seal out infection, plus a spongelike inner layer made of collagen, which replaces the skin's naturally thick, fibrous dermis. The collagen acts as a scaffold for new skin to grow into. The new skin eventually replaces the fake stuff completely as the collagen dissolves. When the process is complete, the artificial epidermis is peeled off and covered with cloned epidermal skin (see page 18) or replaced through other means.

To Nip Colds and Other Bugs . . .

The nagging misery of a cold or the flu is something we all experience from time to time. Here are some quick ways to find relief.

Use "body-regulated" nutrition. Forget "starve a cold and feed a fever." The key to speedy recovery from colds and flus is to feed your body while taking into account what it's telling you, says George Blackburn, M.D., Ph.D., associate professor of surgery at Harvard Medical School and chief of the Nutrition/Metabolism Laboratory at the New England Deaconess Hospital in Boston. If you feel like eating, by all means do so, because your body needs the calories for energy in its battle against whatever may be laying you low. If you don't feel like eating, that's okay, too, Dr. Blackburn says, but only for a period of five days. If you still don't feel like eating after that, try to force yourself, because your body at that point will definitely be running low on its nutritional reserves. And regardless of your appetite for solid foods, always take in plenty of liquids, Dr. Blackburn says. Drink water, juices, or broths to aid the body in its germ warfare.

Exempt from the above five-day rule are people who have been chronically ill, who are underweight, or who are elderly, Dr. Blackburn says. These people should follow a three-day rule—or even less.

Liquidate laryngitis. Good hydration is the fastest way to get rid of a case of laryngitis.

First, make sure you drink plenty of water to keep the larynx itself moist. Ten glasses per day is a good target. The water should be warm—not hot, not cold, no added salt, or alcohol (forget those infamous hot toddies; alcohol is drying). And please, no gargling! It can stress the vocal cords, as does whispering. If you're really hoarse, try to stay as quiet as possible for two days.

Second, suck on hard candies. Almost any flavor will do, including the old standbys of wild cherry, honey, or black currant. Avoid mint or menthol candies, though. They can dry out your vocal cords.

Give yourself the warm-air treatment. From researchers at the Common-Cold Unit at Harvard Hospital in Great Britain comes this good news: Breathing warm, moist air appears to provide immediate relief of cold symptoms.

Cold sufferers made to breathe moist air heated to 109°F for 20 minutes reported symptoms over the next four days that were only half as severe as those of cold sufferers who breathed moist air at room temperature. Relief included less mucus production, nasal congestion, coughing, sore-throat discomfort, and headache pain. But what's the biology behind the relief?

The researchers couldn't say for sure, but they speculate that "heat-shock" genes may play a role, kicking appropriate immunological reactions, including the production of interferon, into gear.

Don't use steam if you're going to try this remedy to gain relief. Steam is far hotter than the 109°F water used in the study and can easily burn the throat and nasal passages.

Put ribavirin to work against childhood pneumonia. Ribavirin is an antiviral prescription drug that clears up the type of pneumonia that occurs in the first three years of life and is caused by respiratory syncytial virus (RSV). It's the only therapy available for this respiratory infection. Some cases clear up on their own, but the infection can become life threatening.

Ribavirin is an aerosol-delivered drug, which means it gets to the lungs instantly. No side effects or tolerance buildup have been reported. And it does hasten the child's recovery.

Ribavirin is currently approved by the Food and Drug Administration (FDA) for RSV-caused lower respiratory tract infections. There is good evidence that it is effective against a number of other viruses, including many common flu bugs, but the FDA has not yet given the green light to these clinical applications.

Fight influenza-A with amantadine. Amantadine is one of a handful of antiviral drugs. It's remarkably effective for reducing the symptoms and duration of flu caused by the influenza-A virus. Doctors recommend the drug for people who are considered at high risk for respiratory infections, such as the elderly and children or people with chronic lung conditions. In fact, it's the only therapy for flu currently approved by the FDA.

Amantadine is taken orally. It's a prescription-only drug, so you need to be diagnosed by a doctor before you can get it. When taken shortly after diagnosis, amantadine relieves aches, fever, and most of the other symptoms of flu.

Use the quickest formula to clear congestion. Winter colds often mean congested chests and endless coughing. The fastest way to clear that congestion is with the nonprescription drug guaifenesin (*gwy-FEN-eh-sin*). In fact, it's the only over-the-counter drug that's approved by the FDA as safe and effective for use as an expectorant.

Because of the FDA ruling, all OTC expectorants that don't contain guaifenesin must be removed from the market and reformulated within a few months.

To Heal Emotional Wounds . . .

No matter what the cause, emotional instability can play havoc with your enjoyment of life. Here are some new ways to get help.

Shed some (fluorescent) light on winter depression. For some it's just a case of the cold-weather grumpies, but for others it becomes a crippling depression—seasonal affective disorder (SAD). It's a darkening of the spirits frequently accompanied by fatigue and weight gain. And it's thought to be caused by a change in brain chemicals brought on by a shortage of sunlight during the winter months. In the past the disorder has been treated with antidepressant drugs, but now encouraging results are being achieved faster with phototherapy—supplying the light the SAD sufferer seems to be missing.

Patients who sit in the vicinity of bright fluorescent light for 2 to 6 hours a day generally notice significant improvement in just two to four days. Antidepressant drugs, which are frequently accompanied by unwanted side effects, can take two weeks or more to bring relief. As much as 20 percent of the U.S. population may suffer from SAD, so phototherapy is currently attracting considerable scientific attention with more and more doctors being trained in administering the treatment.

Recent developments suggest that brighter lighting than that used in previous treatments may be able to shorten exposure times to as little as a half hour a day, with morning thought to be best. You can find more information on SAD and skilled phototherapists, special light-fixture distributors, patient-support, and professional groups in the book *Seasons of the Mind*, by Norman E. Rosenthal, M.D.

Consider time-limited psychotherapy. When some people think of psychotherapy, they think of a doctor/patient relationship that lasts for years. While such long-term treatment may be necessary for some mental illnesses, it's not necessarily the best way to approach more transient problems. So now there's a new trend toward less lengthy psychotherapy that focuses on specific problems rather than everything that's wrong in a person's life.

Time-limited psychotherapy usually extends over 12 to 30 sessions. The patient and therapist set deadlines and goals and discuss the specifics of the patient's problem. There is less of the generalized, "how-did-you-relate-to-your-father" school of soul searching involved.

This approach works best on brief, transient problems, such as divorce, mourning, temporary depression, leaving home for the first time, or troubles at work. The success rate of this approach has been good for many problems. And it can save the patient a lot of money.

The concept of time-limited psychotherapy has spread rapidly. Your doctor or your county mental health office or mental health association may be able to assist you in a search for a professional who uses this approach.

Force yourself to establish routines and continue relationships after the loss of a loved one. Joseph Flaherty, M.D., a professor of psychiatry at the University of Illinois, says that people who do this pull out of the depression following the death of a loved one much faster than people who do not.

The reason, Dr. Flaherty theorizes, is that abrupt change in some people's daily patterns can lead to an abrupt change in biological rhythms, leading to hormonal changes that may foster depression. The hormonal changes can be minimized, he says, if the sense of social upheaval is minimized. Regimentation and social involvement cure depression faster than the martyrdom of trying to go it alone.

To Ease Eye Ills . . .

The laser offers two solutions to vision-threatening conditions.

Ask your doctor about a laser procedure to undo a common complication of cataract surgery. The surgery in question is lens replacement, a procedure in which an artificial lens is implanted in the eye. This now-standard surgery can restore vision to good or near-perfect proficiency. But in about half of all cases the capsule that encloses the lens clouds over. Formerly, another operation was necessary to remove the capsule.

But with the use of a laser, follow-up surgery isn't necessary. The laser doesn't have to burn through anything. Instead, a quick pulse of the laser creates a shock wave in the eye. That makes a tiny hole in the center of the clouded capsule, restoring sight instantly. The patient needs no further treatment or recovery time.

Use the laser against glaucoma. Laser surgery is the fastest way to perform a sight-saving operation on certain glaucoma sufferers. Glaucoma is a potentially serious condition in which fluid buildup causes pressure inside the eye.

Previously, surgery called iridotomy, in which the iris was cut, was the only way to relieve the pressure of acute glaucoma. But the procedure can be done much faster—and more safely and effectively—with a laser. It's now a routine office procedure; the patient can go home on the same day.

To Treat the Feet . . .

When your feet hurt, everything hurts, or so it seems. Here is one way to stop the pain.

Look into one-day, walk-away bunion surgery. Sophisticated surgery combining bioengineering and a single screw has made dreaded bunion surgery something you can walk away from—comfortably. A bunion is a large lump near the ball of the foot. It's caused by bones that shift around behind the big toe. Traditional surgery usually requires four to five days of recuperation in a hospital. The patient has to wear a cast and limit walking for several months. It's not fun.

The new surgery is an outpatient procedure, which means no hospital stay. Most patients are back in normal shoes in three weeks. The secret is a surgical screw that keeps the realigned bones in place after surgery. The patient must go back for follow-up visits, and the screw is removed in a minor procedure four to seven months later. Meanwhile, the patient can get around with little pain or discomfort.

So far, this particular technique is being used only at Medstar Foot and Ankle Center in Sherman Oaks, California (818-784-6231). But there are variations on the procedure being performed in a number of different treatment centers. Ask your podiatrist for a referral.

To Overcome
Gastrointestinal Problems . . .

Here's a summary of the latest developments in treating intestinal distress.

Use ibuprofen for menstrual-related diarrhea. Ordinary ibuprofen (an over-the-counter aspirin substitute) may relieve menstrual-related diarrhea and cramping faster than any other nonprescription drug, says Penny Wise Budoff, M.D., director of the Women's Medical Center in Bethpage, New York. She says her research shows that ibuprofen eases these symptoms by limiting the manufacture of prostaglandins, hormones that cause smooth muscle (as found in the intestines and uterus) to contract. Dr. Budoff says that ibuprofen may also reduce other problems arising during the onset of menstruation, including nausea, vomiting, aching legs, backaches, and headaches.)

The dosage is what you would normally take for pain relief: one or two tablets at the onset of symptoms. Take as often as directed until the symptoms go away. The tablets should be taken with milk or food. (People with ulcers or those who are sensitive to aspirin probably should not use ibuprofen.)

Ask your physician about promising new drugs for inflammatory bowel disease. This category of intestinal disorders includes proctitis, ulcerative colitis, and Crohn's disease and afflicts an estimated 900,000 Americans. In the past, therapy has meant surgery or treatment with drugs known to cause adverse side effects. But scientists now feel encouraged about a new group of drugs that appear to be safer, faster, and more effective.

One such drug that's now available is 5-ASA (brand name Rowasa), which, when administered in enema form, has proved effective in approximately 70 percent of proctitis sufferers who do not respond to cortisone. (Proctitis is characterized by inflammation and bleeding in the lower rectum and is often mistaken for hemorrhoids.) Improvement generally occurs within six to seven weeks when 5-ASA enemas are administered nightly. Because the enemas are quite expensive at $8 each, however, 5-ASA suppositories soon will be available at a reduced cost.

For ulcerative colitis, characterized by inflammation and bleeding of a larger portion of the large intestine than proctitis, 5-ASA can be given in tablet form (Asacol) and taken by mouth. Asacol avoids the side effects of medications containing sulfa or steroids, and it works in roughly

50 to 70 percent of patients. Final FDA approval is expected soon.

Another 5-ASA derivative, called Pentasa, appears to be effective against Crohn's disease (inflammation of the large and small intestine alike) but is yet to be approved by the FDA.

To Zap Gynecological Problems . . .

Women with conditions that jeopardize the chances of pregnancy can be thankful for these new procedures that may help them conceive.

Look into the high-tech remedy for blocked fallopian tubes. Called transcervical balloon tuboplasty (TBT), the procedure involves not surgery, but only a catheter directed through the cervix and uterus to the point of the obstruction. A balloon at the catheter's end is then inflated and the obstruction cleared. In the approximately 70 TBTs done so far, at least one fallopian tube has been successfully cleared in about 90 percent of the women treated. And roughly one-quarter of those women have gone on to become pregnant, reports Edmond Confino, M.D., of the Mount Sinai Hospital Medical Center of Chicago.

Before TBT, microsurgery (which requires general anesthesia and prolonged hospitalization) or *in vitro* fertilization (IVF) were the only ways to achieve pregnancy in patients with fallopian-tube blockage. Microsurgery produces only about a 50 percent success rate, however, and IVF even less than that—about 15 percent. TBT's current success rate for reopening blocked tubes is approximately 90 percent. And coupled with its convenience as an outpatient procedure requiring only local anesthesia, it is a very attractive alternative, Dr. Confino says. For a list of centers offering TBT, contact Dr. Confino at (312) 764-0500.

Consider the new, faster-healing alternative to laparoscopy plus surgery. Nowadays when there's a problem with a woman's reproductive organs, gynecologists often perform a laparoscopy, in which a long, thin tube (called a laparoscope) is used to look around inside the body. The doctor makes a small incision in the abdomen and inserts the laparoscope to see what's the matter. Once the doctor has located the problem, a second surgery may be needed—frequently with a hospital stay. But recently, in treating endometriosis and some cases of infertility, doctors have found a way of doing all this with one procedure. The trick is to use a laser along with the laparoscope. Endometriosis is a painful condition in which uterinelike tissue colonizes other organs in the abdomen and then begins to bleed. It can cause infertility. Scars on the reproductive organs can also cause infertility. A laser shooting through a special laparoscope can vaporize endometrial and scar tissue at the same time the problem is discovered. There is virtually no bleeding, and the minimal operation heals quickly.

To Solve Inner-Ear Problems . . .

Annoying inner-ear conditions can make normal activities difficult. Here are two possible solutions.

Exercise for dizziness relief. Relief from dizziness caused by head injuries or problems with the inner ear can take months. So physical therapists are now speeding the process with special balance-restoring exercises that retrain the central nervous system. After assessing balance difficulties by asking patients to perform such tasks as climbing steps and sitting on a large beach ball, therapists prescribe specific exercises designed to correct what is found. The exercises, which include maneuvers like standing on one foot and walking while turning the head from side to side, are thought to reestablish whatever central nervous system functioning may have been lost.

Therapists feel encouraged that such training may be able to bring relief to people for whom surgery is inappropriate. For more information, check with your physician. He can put you in touch with a center or therapist practicing the techniques. Do not try any such maneuvers on your own, especially if you suffer from heart trouble or arthritis in the neck area.

Consider a new one-day surgery for Meniere's disease. About three years ago, a fairly serious form of surgery was introduced for people with severe vertigo caused by

Meniere's disease, a disorder of the inner ear. In this procedure, one of the nerves in the ear that controls balance is carefully severed, stopping the sending of balance misinformation, thus eliminating the vertigo and halting the slow loss of hearing often found in severe Meniere's. (The other balance-controlling nerve compensates for the loss.) But the surgery was still surgery—requiring a week or two of recuperation in a hospital.

In a new procedure, the doctor makes an incision behind the ear and places a capsule of streptomycin directly on the balance organ. Streptomycin is an antibiotic that's able to destroy the sensory cells in the balance-controlling nerve, achieving the same result as the traditional surgery. After the incision is sewn up, the patient can go home. And as with the older kind of surgery, whatever hearing remains is preserved. Experts expect that the procedure will be available soon at several medical centers.

To Hurry Healing without Surgery . . .

Here's the latest on some new procedures that may help you avoid major surgery.

Shrink hemorrhoids with infrared light. Great advances have been made in hemorrhoid therapy, but the best of all may be infrared photocoagulation—a procedure that shrinks hemorrhoids in seconds with bursts of infrared light delivered via a fiberoptic probe. It's nearly painless, causes very little bleeding, involves no risk of infection, usually requires no anesthesia and can be done on an outpatient basis, with patients being up and about immediately following the 5- to 10-minute procedure.

The technique also allows several hemorrhoids to be treated in a single procedure, unlike rubber-band ligation, which allows just one hemorrhoid to be treated at a time. Cost of the technique also is a huge plus—roughly one-quarter to one-fifth the price of surgery.

Colon and rectal surgeon John O'Connor, M.D., of Suburban Hospital in Bethesda, Maryland, says photocoagulation is appropriate for approximately 50 to 60 percent of the hemorrhoid sufferers he sees who need treatment. It's an especially good choice for pregnant women because it injects nothing into the bloodstream, Dr. O'Connor says. It is not, however, suitable for hemorrhoids that protrude outside the anus. These external hemorrhoids usually require surgery.

Photocoagulation is now being widely practiced, so check with a gastroenterologist or rectal and colon surgeon in your area for someone competent in the technique.

Ask about lasers for undoing the complications of kidney stone lithotripsy. Sonic shock-wave lithotripsy has become a standard treatment for kidney stones. In this painless procedure, sound waves bombard and break up the stones, with no scalpel required. But sometimes all does not go well: The stones do break up, but large pieces get stuck in the ureter as they are being passed. The pieces lodge in an area of the body where it is difficult and dangerous to perform lithotripsy. Surgery—the very thing lithotripsy was supposed to replace—was the only answer. Until now. The faster answer requires a laser and a fiberoptic thread contained in a long tube called a ureteroscope. The scope is snaked up to the blockage, and the laser is fired in short pulses. It forms a shock wave that breaks up the kidney stone fragment into passable pieces. The patient can go home the same day in most cases. The procedure is safe, effective, and best of all, quicker than nature or the knife. For now, laser lithotripsy is limited to several large centers in the United States. Consult your physician.

Zap brain tumors safely with new pinpoint radiation. A new technique can destroy small brain tumors and abnormally formed blood vessels without making an incision in the skull. And when you don't cut open the skull, the patient heals much, much faster than after ordinary surgery.

The patient lies on a surgical table with his head immobilized in a metal ring. The surgical team plots the location of the tumor or blood vessel in relation to the ring by using a CAT scanner or magnetic imaging device. Once the target is located, the patient is moved under a special x-ray machine mounted to a rotating turret. The machine shoots a precise x-ray beam at the patient's head, through the target area. The turret rotates slightly as it continuously beams radiation from different angles. The procedure continues for about 30 minutes.

The patient feels nothing. And the tumor or vessels receive a cumulative dose of radiation, while the surrounding tissue has received a very minimal dose. In the case of a tumor, the tissue dies and scars over in a few weeks to months. Blood vessel abnormalities can take up to two or three years to completely disappear.

But in either case, usually no further treatment is needed.

Of course, the equipment needed for this procedure is very expensive and not yet widely available. Johns Hopkins Medical Institutions is one of the top centers now performing this knifeless surgery. For information on other centers, call Johns Hopkins at (301) 955-2259.

To Fight Back against Heart Problems . . .

Heart patients may benefit from these new techniques and treatments.

Ensure faster absorption of nitroglycerin tablets for angina relief. You can do this with a simple squirt of salt water beneath the tongue, reports Frank E. Rasler, M.D., in the *New England Journal of Medicine*. Adequate moisture is needed for prompt absorption of nitroglycerin by the mouth tissue, Dr. Rasler says, but saliva can tend to be in short supply due to apprehension and altered breathing during an angina attack. Simply by dousing beneath the tongue with about ¼ teaspoon of salt water, however, moisture can quickly be restored. "This simple action has frequently resulted in prompt relief of pain when previous doses of nitroglycerin . . . had failed," Dr. Rasler reports.

A nitroglycerin spray also is now available to circumvent the dry mouth syndrome. It enjoys the additional advantage over tablets of being easier to administer for elderly patients who may have trouble opening tablet containers. The spray also boasts a shelf life of approximately three years, compared to the three- to six-month period of effectiveness for nitroglycerin in tablet form.

With your doctor's okay, work out for a faster post-

heart-attack recovery. Doctors used to be reluctant to allow patients to do anything strenuous for several months after a heart attack. Current wisdom states that a moderate program of aerobic activity—walking, biking, swimming, and the like—is the best and fastest way to get back to normal. And in many cases, the patient can begin some activity within a few days after hospital discharge. Of course, the final decision concerning post-heart-attack activity rests with the doctor. Most sufferers of "simple" heart attack and even those who are recovering from heart attack complications can benefit from exercise.

Let clot-busting drugs spare the heart muscle. Streptokinase, a drug that dissolves blood clots, can speed healing by limiting the amount of heart-muscle damage that occurs just after a heart attack. It works only if the heart attack is caused by a blood clot blocking off a coronary artery that has been narrowed by cholesterol buildup. But it's remarkably effective if it's given to the patient as soon as possible after the first sign of heart attack—in time to prevent large areas of heart muscle from being starved of oxygen.

Two more expensive drugs are used from time to time for the same purpose: urokinase and tissue-type plasminogen activator (t-PA). Streptokinase is currently the drug of choice, according to several researchers.

To Turn Off Pain . . .

Runners, take heed. Here's how to fight a common complaint.

Breathe through runner's cramps. The fastest way to relieve painful side stitches while jogging is to breathe slowly and rhythmically. Often these cramps are caused by spasms of the overworked diaphragm, the muscle that helps expand and contract your lungs. By breathing slowly and rhythmically—and slowing your pace—you can work through the cramp.

To Unclog Sinuses . . .

Here's a recent development in surgery that can speed recovery.

See about faster-healing sinus surgery. For standard sinus surgery, doctors cut through and around the bones of the upper face. But some surgeons have perfected the technique of endoscopic intranasal sinus surgery: opening the sinuses by reaching up through the nose with special instruments under the guidance of a small telescope. This new surgery helps surgeons limit trauma during the procedure; therefore, patients heal faster afterward. In this surgery, the surgeon can see with greater accuracy what needs to be done and can remove only enough tissue to open the sinuses properly.

Although it was introduced to this country from Europe only about five years ago, endoscopic intranasal surgery for sinus blockage seems to be gaining popularity with surgeons, according to Stanley M. Shapshay, M.D., chairman of the Department of Otolaryngology (head and neck surgery) at the Lahey Clinic in Burlington, Massachusetts. Check with the nearest university or teaching hospital if you are interested in the procedure.

To Smooth Out Skin Problems . . .

From eczema to birthmarks to acne, researchers are discovering more effective treatments for skin conditions.

Use antiscratching therapy to speed the healing of eczema. Eczema (atopic dermatitis) is a problem not only because it causes dry, flaking skin but also because it itches, which prompts scratching that only makes the condition worse. A standard therapy is hydrocortisone cream. In a Swedish study, though, eczema patients were instructed in how to resist the scratching urge and saw significantly greater improvements from hydrocortisone cream application than patients who were given the cream but no instructions.

Antiscratching therapy was given in two sessions. The first taught patients to press firmly on the affected area for 1 minute whenever they felt the urge to scratch, and then to move their hands to their thighs or to an object. The second session instructed the patients to avoid the affected area entirely; they were told to move their hands to their thighs or to grasp an object directly. Results: After four weeks, patients given the antiscratch therapy plus cream had nearly twice the improvement of the patients given the cream but no therapy.

"Any treatment program for . . . eczema should include steps to reduce scratching," concluded the doctors in their *British Journal of Dermatology* report.

Laser away port-wine stain birthmarks. The new "tunable dye" laser is the preferred device to use when removing a type of birthmark known as a port-wine stain. The birthmark, which usually appears as a reddish or purple blotch on the face or neck, is caused by an overabundance of blood vessels near the surface of the skin. The light of the laser can be "tuned" to the precise wavelength that's best absorbed by a particular birthmark. As the vessels absorb the light, they heat up and, in a sense, self-destruct. The process leaves little or no scarring.

Before lasers, there were no good surgical options for port-wine stain removal. The argon laser was the first device used on these birthmarks, but it left a more noticeable scar. The tunable dye laser procedure may take several office visits before the treatment is complete. Almost all port-wine stains can be altered dramatically, and some can be totally cleared. It's an outpatient procedure each time—no hospital stay is required. For adult patients, it's a relatively painless procedure as well. The after-procedure sensation has been compared to a sunburn.

Check out retinoic acid. It's a form of vitamin A that can speed healing in certain skin conditions. It works best as a topically applied gel or cream for the reversal of sun damage (including wrinkles) and to clear up severe acne. There are indications that retinoic acid may have a broader healing scope, and research is under way. Don't be fooled by nonprescription sound-alikes, such as retinol or retinoids (beta-carotene). Retinoic acid is a prescription-only drug. It should be used only under the care of a physician.

Try a new antibiotic gel for adult acne. For people who don't get relief from standard oral antibiotics, it's better and faster. Although teenagers have a choice of dozens of medications for "common" acne, people suffering from adult acne (rosacea, pronounced *row-ZAY-she-uh*) used to have only one option: oral antibiotics, usually tetracycline. Over time, this therapy can have undesirable side effects (for example, the decimation of beneficial bacteria in the intestine). And in many cases, oral antibiotics just aren't very effective.

But the new topical gel is a prescription drug (brand name: MetroGel) containing metronidazole (*meh-troh-NYE-dah-zole*), a powerful antibiotic that's difficult to tolerate in oral doses. When rubbed directly on skin, it's virtually free of side effects. In clinical tests, metronidazole gel reduced rosacea inflammation rapidly during the first three weeks of therapy, achieving maximum results by the ninth week.

Metronidazole gel won't give everyone with rosacea a completely clear face in three weeks. Right now, nothing is 100 percent effective for everybody. But it does provide a significant reduction in the disease faster and better than anything else. Ask your dermatologist about it.

To Get a Better Night's Sleep . . .

Ah, sleep, glorious sleep! If it's only a dream for you, check out this advice.

Check your minerals. A quick and healthy way to improve the quality of your sleep might be to make sure that you're getting enough copper and iron in your diet, suggests new research by James G. Penland, Ph.D., of the USDA Human Nutrition Research Center at Grand Forks, North Dakota. Dr. Penland found that when women's intake of these trace minerals was reduced to roughly one-third of recommended amounts, their sleep suffered in significant and measurable ways. Reduced iron intake resulted in an increase in the number of awakenings during the night, while reduced copper resulted in an increase in time taken to fall asleep.

So if the most common culprits in insomnia have been ruled out (like stress, too much physical activity just before bedtime, or alcohol use), be sure that your copper and iron intakes are up to snuff. (Serious, chronic insomnia, of course, needs a doctor's attention.)

To get the U.S. Recommended Daily Allowance

(USRDA) of copper (2 milligrams), look to copper-rich foods, such as liver (one slice has 2.4 milligrams), oysters (2.75 milligrams per ¼ cup), tofu (1 cup has 0.97 milligram), and refried beans (1 milligram per cup). Supplementation with copper can be dangerous because levels as low as 10 to 12 milligrams can be toxic.

To achieve the iron USRDA of 18 milligrams a day, eat iron-rich sources, such as red meat (5.12 milligrams in a 6-ounce sirloin), clams (one serving has 11.9 milligrams), and garbanzo beans (13.8 milligrams per 1 cup, dried). Menstruating women, people on restricted diets, pregnant and lactating women, and a few others are at risk for iron deficiency. They should check with their doctor about supplements.

To Bounce Back after Surgery . . .

Many factors influence how quickly patients recover after an operation. Here are a few ways to stack the deck in your favor.

Look into patches for hernia repair. A synthetic patch is making hernia repair virtually a one-day outpatient procedure. Standard stitch-'em-up hernia surgery usually requires a postsurgical hospital stay of several days, followed by weeks of convalescence and limited activity. "But the patch works so well that many patients can go back to work the next day," says Irving L. Lichtenstein, M.D., director of the Lichtenstein Hernia Institute.

A hernia is a tear in the muscle fiber of the abdomen—not unlike a tear in fabric. When it's sewed up the regular way, there is tension on the edges of the tear during movement. But when a patch is sewn over the tear, tension is eliminated because the edges of the tear aren't being pulled back together. At the same time, the tear can't get any bigger because the patch holds it in place.

The patch is a mesh web made of Marlex, a polypropylene plastic. It's not rejected by the body as a foreign substance. Quite the opposite, in fact: It acts as a scaffold for new tissue growth.

The patch procedure for hernia repair has been used by

some surgeons for over 20 years. It was originally conceived for people with recurrent hernias, but it's been found safe and extremely effective for all hernia cases. It hasn't been widely adopted yet, but more surgeons have been learning this procedure in recent years.

Listen to some tunes. Studies by music therapist Helen Lindquist Bonny, Ph.D., suggest that surgery patients experience lower blood pressure and reduced heart rates while treated to soothing classical music before their operations. She says that they also need less pain medication and are able to leave the hospital sooner when exposed to more tunes after their surgeries. "The right music can create both a situation of relaxation for surgery patients prior to their ordeals and a diversion from pain afterward," Dr. Bonny says.

Before asking to be treated to Led Zeppelin while being rolled into the operating room (OR), however, understand that music should be of "regular rhythm, and have predictable dynamics and consonance of harmony" to work its soothing wonders, Dr. Bonny says. For that reason, she recommends that patients consult a music therapist before deciding on their surgical selections.

Ask the surgeon about "surgical glue." When surgeons can't use stitches, they use adhesives. And one of the most promising new surgical adhesives comes from doctors at the University of Pennsylvania. The glue speeds healing because it's more compatible with the patient's own tissues than synthetic glues.

Called "autologous fibrinogen adhesive," the glue is composed of natural compounds (fibrin and thrombin) that are responsible for the clotting of the blood. When these two components are combined, they solidify in approximately 2 minutes, forming an artificial clot that helps hold tissue in place. The clot also gives cells something to cling to as they proliferate, thus greatly assisting and accelerating the healing process. The adhesive then gets absorbed harmlessly by the body as healing progresses.

Thus far the procedure has proved most effective in situations where tissue is not subjected to much postoperative stress, such as in surgeries of the inner ear, microsurgeries, and nerve repairs. The adhesive is showing great promise, reports Leslie Silberstein, M.D., of the Hospital of the University of Pennsylvania, but still remains in experimental stages.

Ask for a hospital roommate who has successfully undergone major surgery. Then you, too, may be likely to recover more quickly from your own surgery. Sound crazy? Not according to a small study from the University of California at San Diego. The study of 27 coronary-bypass patients tested two variables: (1) whether the roommate was awaiting or recovering from surgery and (2) whether the roommate underwent the same operation or a different procedure.

Consistently, the patients who roomed with someone who was recovering from surgery did better than patients who roomed with someone awaiting surgery. They were far less anxious before their operation. Afterward, they were more physically active, presumably from having observed the recovery of the experienced roommate. In the end, they were released from the hospital an average of 1.4 days earlier than patients who roomed with a person awaiting surgery. As it turned out, it didn't matter what kind of surgery the roommate had had, as long as it was a major procedure. The authors of the study acknowledge the need for more data (it's not wise to make recommendations for everyone based on a 27-person study), but their findings are practical and wouldn't cost anything extra to implement.

Destress yourself before surgery. Learning how to lighten your load psychologically before going into the operating room may help you recover faster, says Notre Dame psychologist George Howard, Ph.D. Dr. Howard found that surgical patients recovered an average of 3½ days faster than a control group if they were first taught how to deal with the mental stress their operations would involve. These destressed patients also experienced less pain and required less pain medication. They also were rated by their nurses as more cooperative in their attitude.

The antistress techniques included deep breathing, muscle relaxation, and thinking soothing thoughts.

Why would these strategies affect recovery? Dr. Howard speculates that the amount of energy available for physical healing is greater when we don't waste energy dealing with psychological stress. The relaxed mind draws less on the reserves needed by the healing body.

Dr. Howard says that anyone who is interested in learning stress-relieving techniques should check with a licensed clinician specializing in pain reduction or anxiety management.

Consider arthroscopy, an alternative to conventional joint surgery. As many as 800,000 of these operations may now be performed each year, and for good reason. Recovery times from arthroscopy can be as short as one or two weeks, compared to six weeks or longer for an equivalent joint operation performed via standard surgery.

Arthroscopy (from *arthro,* meaning joint, and *scope,* meaning to see) avoids the disadvantages of standard cut-and-stitch surgery thanks to a thin telescope that relays color pictures to an operating-room monitor. The surgeon makes a much smaller incision (resulting in less trauma to the patient) and inserts the telescope.

Using smaller-than-normal instruments, the surgeon is then able to diagnose and/or do repair work according to what he sees magnified on the screen.

Though used most often on knees, the procedure also can be applied to shoulders, elbows, ankles, wrists, and even the jaw in the case of temporomandibular joint (TMJ) dysfunction. The technique is even being used on joint infections, arthritis, and joint injuries. Arthroscopy is usually performed on an outpatient basis, with only local rather than general anesthesia required.

If appropriate, opt for lasers instead of scalpels. Lasers have single-handedly reduced healing time in a variety of standard surgical procedures. A laser beam can cut more precisely than the blade of a scalpel, which means less damage to surrounding tissue. The beam cauterizes blood vessels as it cuts, so less blood is lost during surgery. And there's less chance of infection because in most cases nothing enters the incision except the laser's light. All these factors make laser-surgery wounds heal better and faster than wounds arising from standard surgeries.

True, lasers can be expensive and may not be the best choice for all surgeries. But many simple laser procedures can be done on an outpatient basis. That's not just quicker healing—that's money saved by eliminating the cost of a hospital stay.

To Cope with Vein Problems . . .

Although artery-clogging plaque can be serious and varicose veins may be only a cosmetic concern, there are new ways to relieve both.

Sand away some types of artery blockage. A device that actually sands down plaque blockage in the arteries is now available on a limited basis. The device, called a rotablator, is tiny and attaches to a spaghetti-thin catheter—like the type used for another artery-opening operation, balloon angioplasty. But in balloon angioplasty, the balloon merely compacts plaque against the vessel wall, then stretches the vessel wall. The rotablator "sands" the plaque off into tiny particles that are carried away in the bloodstream.

At this writing, the rotablator is being used experimentally at several medical centers around the country. While the rotablator isn't perfect for every kind of plaque blockage, says Robert Ginsburg, M.D., director of the Center for Advanced Cardiovascular Therapy at Stanford University Medical Center, it's probably the most promising of several types of devices currently under investigation.

One of the best features of the rotablator is that it leaves a smoother surface than other devices. That probably will translate into a lower reblockage rate, although that's one of the things research should determine. Like balloon angioplasty, the rotablator procedure can be done in a few minutes to hours, with the patient able to leave the next day. That's because only a small incision is required to get the catheter into the artery.

Consider the "instant" varicose vein remover. Would you believe a treatment for varicose veins that makes them disappear right before your eyes? No, it's not magic. It's sclerotherapy, the nonsurgical alternative to vein-stripping surgery for smaller secondary veins.

For many years, the only way to get rid of "road-map legs" was to have the veins removed through such surgery—a painful procedure with some risk of complications. Sclerotherapy is not a form of surgery, so there are no incisions to heal. A saline solution is injected into the vein, irritating it to the point where it shrivels up and closes off. On smaller "spider" veins, the effect is quite dramatic: You can watch the vein "disappear" as the saline displaces the blood. Over the next one to three months, the vein breaks down and is absorbed by the body. But for cosmetic purposes, the vein fades within minutes of the procedure.

People who've undergone sclerotherapy report a mild burning sensation during and shortly after the injection. The worst side effect? Some patients suffer a tiny, temporary skin ulcer or a frecklelike mark near the injection site. All patients are able to walk away from the procedure, although strenuous activity is discouraged for a day.

To Speed Wound Healing . . .

For cuts, scrapes, and other injuries, here's some speedy first aid.

Try the newfangled antibiotic ointments. They can knock four days off the healing time of a minor cut or scrape. Unfortunately, many people still simply fall back on their grandma's favorite antiseptic remedy, such as iodine or peroxide. But doing that could be worse than doing nothing at all, according to a study.

Two different antibiotic ointments were tested against a variety of "traditional" antiseptic treatments, including iodine, hydrogen peroxide, and Mercurochrome. In the interests of science, 47 volunteers submitted to six minor wounds (three on each arm), which were later infected with a mild strain of staphylococcus. One wound out of every six was left untreated to act as a control.

Each untreated wound healed by itself in an average of 13 days. Both a dual antibiotic ointment (polymyxin B/bacitracin) and a triple antibiotic (neomycin/polymyxin B/bacitracin) healed wounds in an average of nine days—that's more than 25 percent faster. None of the antiseptic preparations speeded wound healing—some even slowed healing time down to an average of 16 days.

Why were multiple antibiotics better? Antiseptics kill

bacteria, but they also kill innocent bystanders: the skin cells that are trying to regrow. Broad-spectrum antibiotic ointments kill bacteria without damaging the healing tissue.

Try the sugar solution. Research has revealed the effectiveness of applying sugar to bedsores and other hard-to-heal wounds—a remedy that has been around since the seventeenth century. The treatment can dramatically speed the healing process in these more serious wounds. (It's not for minor cuts and scrapes.) By absorbing moisture from the wounds, the sugar forms a concentrated solution that creates an unfavorable environment for bacterial growth, says *Prevention* adviser Alvin B. Segelman, Ph.D., professor of pharmacognosy at Rutgers University College of Pharmacy.

Sugar also acts as a kind of scavenger, picking up dead bacteria and white blood cells. This debris then can be easily flushed away when the wound is gently washed with warm salt water.

Because all serious wounds (including bedsores and diabetic ulcers) should be under the care of a physician, sugar treatments should be applied under medical supervision. The sugar treatment is not a home remedy, cautions Dr. Segelman.

Check with your doctor about a new treatment for venous ulcers. Skin ulcers caused by blood clots in the veins of the legs heal twice as fast when treated with a new antiseptic known as cadexomer iodine, according to a study of 54 patients reported in the *Western Journal of Medicine*. Compared to ulcers treated with the standard methods of gauze bandages soaked in salt water, ulcers treated once daily with cadexomer iodine healed from 1½ to 2½ times faster. Trends toward less pain and less swelling also were observed with the new antiseptic. The only drawbacks appeared to be mild burning or itching experienced by 6 of the 38 cadexomer iodine patients.

The researchers theorize that the cadexomer iodine (which goes on in a powdered form) draws fluid from the ulcers, and with that fluid, much of the infection-causing bacteria. The iodine also helps kill the bacteria.

Take advantage of your blood's own medicine. Growth factors harvested from platelets—the substance in blood that helps form clots—can speed healing of skin ulcers and other wounds that don't heal on their own. Growth factors are specialized proteins that can trigger cells to divide and grow. Platelet-derived growth factors are only one of many similar substances produced by our bodies.

David Knighton, M.D., director of the wound-healing program at the University of Minnesota Hospital, has developed an economical method of extracting growth factors from the blood of each patient. Only 2 ounces (about 4 tablespoons) of blood are needed to produce the necessary amount. The growth factors are then applied directly to the wound. Since the patient gets only the growth factors extracted from his or her own blood, there is no chance of contracting a blood-borne disease, such as AIDS or hepatitis. Right now, Dr. Knighton's method is used primarily on people with diabetic and other nonhealing skin ulcers within a comprehensive wound-care program. (It may be useful for burn patients, too.) It's not economical to use on ordinary wounds because most heal on their own with a natural, blood-borne dose of these same growth factors. For information on availability, call the Curatech company at (800) 544-2572.

Seal the wound airtight. Forget the old advice about "letting the air get at it." Keeping a cut moist with an occlusive (airtight) dressing can help it heal as much as 40 percent faster than using gauze or other bandages. Doctors aren't certain exactly why this speeds healing. One theory states that an occlusive dressing keeps healing substances in body fluids from evaporating. But no matter what the mechanism, it works.

On the market there are several types of brand-name occlusive dressing made of polyurethane film. The slightly different hydrocolloid dressings have polyurethane exteriors with an interior layer of biocompatible material that "melts" into the wound. Hydrogel dressings are made of water and polyethylene oxide. The best-known of these is Spenco's 2nd Skin (for information, call 800-433-3334).

Occlusive dressings may not be ideal for chronic

wounds, such as diabetic ulcers. That's because there's an underlying problem (for example, diabetes) that retards natural healing. But for most minor cuts, an occlusive dressing is best.

Apply heat. Open wounds or muscle strains are likely to heal faster if the area is heated slightly, reports John Rabkin, M.D., an instructor in surgery at the University of California at San Francisco.

In a review of several studies, Dr. Rabkin hypothesizes that heat dilates the blood vessels in the area of an injury, which increases blood flow and hence the influx of oxygen. Oxygen in turn seems to accelerate the production of collagen, a crucial element in the healing process.

Try applying heat in the form of a heating pad; hot-water bottle; or warm, moist towel in a plastic bag for 15 to 30 minutes, four to six times a day.

Applying heat first, however, does not work on sprains or ligament injuries.

Sprains and ligament problems should probably be allowed to have their swelling subside (by using ice on them) before heat is applied, but heat may then be used in the same manner as with open wounds, Dr. Rabkin says. (Of course, any serious injury should get a doctor's attention.)

The only people who should not use heat therapy are those with neuropathy (nerve damage). They may not be able to feel if the heat they're applying is too extreme and may burn themselves as a result.

CHAPTER 4

Medical Mimics

Drugs that regulate the body's healing and growth processes open a new frontier.

For Jill Jones, life before the age of biotechnology was an endless round of illnesses.

The Brighton, Michigan, teenager has a rare, life-threatening blood disorder called neutropenia, a shortage of infection-fighting white blood cells. The little ailments of daily life—colds, sore throats, ear infections—could send her to the hospital. At times, her mouth sores were so painful that she couldn't eat. She tried attending college but left after a few months; sickness struck so often that continuing was pointless.

Then in February 1989, Jones was chosen to take part in experiments with a new bioengineered drug aimed at bolstering her body's natural defenses. Her father wept.

After several months on the drug, Jones, 19, was able to begin leading a life approaching that of a normal teen-ager. She can at last focus on the little *pleasures* of daily life—a trip out of town with a friend, a night of dancing. She is once again planning to enroll in college. For the first time in years, she says, "I have felt really good. It's wonderful."

Jones is a pioneer on biotechnology's hottest new frontier: the development of man-made "growth factors," drugs that mimic the body's natural proteins that regulate the growth and healing processes of cells. For years, scientists have known about the powerful role played by these scarce proteins. Now biotechnology's ability to produce them holds out the promise of a medical revolution.

Broken Bones and Burns

Already, scientists are testing growth factors on humans in hopes of treating ulcers, burns, broken bones, and the often-devastating side effects of cancer and AIDS treatments. Others hope growth factors will one day reverse some of the chronic degenerative ailments of old age, including heart disease, arthritis, and osteoporosis.

"We're seeing the real fruits of the biotechnology revolution," says Jerome Groopman, a leader in testing growth factors at Boston's New England Deaconess Hospital. "It really is a new era in medicine." The growing availability of the potent proteins, adds Andrew Baird, a biochemist at the Whittier Institute for Diabetes and Endocrinology at La Jolla, California, means that "we can seriously sit down and think of things that existed only in science fiction before."

The new era, however, is just dawning; most of the drugs are still years from the market. Only one of the new growth factors—erythropoietin (EPO), which stimulates production of red blood cells—has been approved by the Food and Drug Administration for routine use in patients. Other blood-stimulating substances, including Neupogen, the Amgen, Inc. drug that is being taken by Jill Jones, are still in clinical trials. Human tests of bone-growth substances are just beginning, and nerve-growth factors are still in early animal trials.

Moreover, it isn't clear yet that scientists can make broad improvements in the body's natural responses to disease, injury, and aging. The blood-cell stimulators are by far the simplest growth factors. The healing process in other tissues, such as skin, bones, and nerves, is much more complex. "There are a lot of hurdles to be met," says Dr. Baird.

Researchers need a better understanding of the growth factors' role in causing or preventing cancer, for instance, before they can eliminate the risk that they will spin out of control. The growth factor boom also raises a serious cost issue: Many of these drugs would have to be taken repeatedly—some for life—and the expense may be enormous.

Fewer Transfusions

Clearly, though, the drugs already have the ability to vastly improve the quality of life for many people. Consider EPO. The drug, which analysts estimate will have sales of more than $500 million within a few years, cures anemia in some patients and in others eliminates the need for blood transfusions.

For years, John Cole, a Lorain, Ohio, newspaper editor with kidney disease, suffered worsening anemia caused by regular dialysis treatments. He needed weekly transfusions that haunted him with the fear of contracting AIDS, and he felt so drained that he could barely drag himself to work.

"Taking out the trash was a major undertaking," he says; a walk on the beach with his wife was out of the question. After 2½ years on EPO, Cole, 40, no longer needs transfusions, his anemia is under control, and he works out three times a week. "I feel tremendous," he says.

EPO also is expected to help patients store their own blood in anticipation of surgery by raising their bodies' red blood-cell production. Teena L. Lerner, a biotechnology analyst at Shearson Lehman Hutton, Inc., estimates that EPO could reduce the need for transfusions from others by 20 percent by 1993.

Close behind in clinical trials are white-cell stimulators, including Neupogen and related products under development by Genetics Institute, Inc., Cambridge, Massschusetts, and Immunex Corporation, Seattle, in marketing partnerships with pharmaceutical firms.

The substances seem certain to improve survival prospects for some cancer patients. While chemotherapy effectively kills cancer cells, it also kills the bone marrow that produces infection-fighting white blood cells, forcing doctors to reduce or halt chemotherapy treatments. Only an estimated 20 percent of the one million patients who undergo chemotherapy each year receive the full prescribed, or target, amount.

The blood-cell growth factors can combat the toxic side effects, some clinical trials show, helping to restore the white cells to normal levels after chemotherapy. That significantly reduces the risk of infections and frees the physician to administer target doses of chemotherapy.

"It's exciting," says Jeffrey Crawford, who has seen the drug improve the condition of lung cancer patients undergoing chemotherapy in clinical trials at Duke University Medical Center and the Durham, North Carolina, Veterans Administration Medical Center. "It takes away some of the obstacles we've had, in terms of what we can do for patients."

Rejected Marrow

Another white-cell–stimulating factor nearly doubled the short-term survival rate of cancer patients who had rejected transplanted bone marrow, a common and often fatal event following chemotherapy or radiation treatments for cancer. The drug has also been shown to bolster white-cell levels in patients with AIDS, enabling some to tolerate treatment with the antiviral drug AZT.

Other growth factors show promise in healing wounds. More than 60 papers on such growth factors have been published in the last five years, according to the *New England Journal of Medicine*. The growing availability of the proteins "has swept aside medicine's traditionally cautious attitude toward the acceleration of healing," the journal reported in an editorial.

In one test with burn patients, a skin-healing agent called epidermal growth factor (EGF) shortened by about a day and a half the time needed to heal wounds created in skin-grafting operations. Chiron Corp. of Emeryville, California, will soon begin testing EGF for healing eye tissue after cataract surgery. Chiron is testing EGF for treating severe stomach ulcers.

Scientists are also in hot pursuit of substances designed to heal or rebuild bone. International Genetic Engineering, Inc., Santa Monica, California, is beginning human trials of a bone growth substance it calls osteogenic factor. In animal experiments, the protein helped repair cranial and limb injuries in rats and rabbits in three to five weeks. Eventually, the substance might be used to repair severe limb fractures, deformed cranial and facial bones, or jaw-bones damaged by periodontal disease, says Arup Sen, executive vice-president of International Genetic Engineering.

The research is increasingly ambitious, focusing on broad-acting, more complex growth factors that affect more than one kind of tissue or even the entire metabolism. Genentech, Inc. has begun human trials of a highly active protein, insulin-like growth factor I, for a condition called wasting syndrome, in which seriously ill or injured patients begin to lose lean muscle tissue and their ability to use the food they eat. Chiron has begun testing the same substance for use in treating osteoporosis, a thinning of bones.

"You're talking about an area of molecular biology that's

moving at an incredible pace" says Paul Reier, a neuroscientist at the University of Florida in Gainesville.

Progress, though, has a price. Epogen, Amgen's brand name for EPO, costs about $4,000 to $8,000 a year, depending on the patient's weight. While Neupogen hasn't been priced yet, some patients are already worried about the cost. "You're not going to see low-priced drugs coming out of this research," says Shearson's Lerner.

Hurdles for Scientists

The field also presents some novel hurdles for medical science. For instance, blood growth factors can easily be injected, and bandages, gels, and lotions can be used to hold wound-healing agents in place. But applying the substances to bones or nerves is a far more difficult matter. "The big problem with growth factor biology today is delivery," says the Whittier Institute's Dr. Baird.

Bruce Pharriss, senior vice-president, science and technology, for Collagen Corp., a Palo Alto, California, biotechnology concern, adds, "We have to find a way to have the stuff in high concentrations in the tissues that need it, and low concentration in those that don't."

Many growth factors are dizzyingly complex, raising further concerns about unforeseen side effects. Many play multiple roles in the body. One promising agent called fibroblast growth factor, for instance, prevents the death of nerve cells in laboratory cultures as well as stimulates healing of cartilage in animal experiments.

Other growth factors react differently in different settings. One protein, called transforming growth factor beta, retards capillary growth in the laboratory but stimulates it in laboratory animals. The factors "are like symbols of the alphabet. They mean one thing in one context and something else in another," says Michael B. Sporn, a leading growth factor researcher at the National Cancer Institute.

Some of the substances have had startling side effects in clinical trials; one blood growth factor unexpectedly reduced cholesterol levels in patients.

Eventually, such unforeseen effects "may lead to new

therapeutic ideas," Marcus Reidenberg, a Cornell University Medical Center physician, wrote in the *Journal of the American Medical Association*. There's evidence, for instance, that some of the blood-cell factors play a role in causing leukemia; researchers hope to harness them in a way that will reverse the disease.

For heart attack victims, applying a growth factor to damaged cardiac tissue following a heart attack might help the organ repair itself, Dr. Sporn suggests. The same factor is believed to curb the body's immune responses under some circumstances, raising hopes that it might be used to treat such chronic inflammatory diseases as rheumatoid arthritis.

Neurologists are peering still further into the growth factor frontier, setting their sights on spinal cord or brain tissue repair. Jerry Silver, a neuroscientist at Case Western Reserve University in Cleveland, has had some success in restoring severed nerves in rats and cats by implanting nerve tissue from embryos; other scientists are claiming success in working with nerve growth factor, a protein found in many parts of the nervous system, to regenerate damaged tissue. "I think there's hope" that, eventually, "we can cure spinal cord injury or massive stroke" victims, Dr. Silver says.

Ultimately, scientists may seek to regulate every cell of the body, yielding "a vast array of products, most of which probably haven't been discovered yet," says David Stone, a spokesman for Genetics Institute. The field, he says, "represents a large part of the potential of biotechnology."

CHAPTER 5

Unheralded Healers from Nature Offer Hope

Substances from land and sea show promise against ovarian cancer, pain, bone breakdown, and more.

Not so long ago, if you told people that oil from certain kinds of fish may lower heart attack risks, they'd respond in one of three ways: (1) "That's insane." (2) "What should I do, rub it on my chest?" (3) "Sounds pretty fishy. [Laughing hysterically.] Get it?" Which just goes to show how today's you've-got-to-be-kidding experiments can become tomorrow's we-knew-it-all-along treatments.

With this in mind, here are eight of today's most intriguing and offbeat remedies. Some have been used with preliminary success in humans. Others have only test-tube or animal tests to back them up. So you may not be able to get your hands on all of them yet, but we think you'll find them interesting just the same.

It'll be a while before the medical world knows for sure if they'll pan out, but they seem clearly worth the wait.

Curing with Frog Slime?

Kiss a frog and you won't get a prince—but you might get a small dose of magainin (*mah-GAY-nin*), an infection-fighting substance that a few people speculate could turn out to be the penicillin of the 1990s.

Magainin (named after the Hebrew word for shield) was discovered by Michael A. Zasloff, M.D., Ph.D., while he was performing genetic research on the eggs of African clawed frogs at the National Institutes of Health. After harvesting the eggs, he sewed up each frog and returned it to an aquarium filled with murky water, similar to the frog's natural habitat. In time, he noticed that none of the frogs developed infections in their rather unsterile environment.

In fact, the frogs' wounds healed quite nicely in about four weeks, with no signs of a normal infection-fighting response (inflammation, pus, and other signs). Dr. Zasloff theorized that some unique type of antimicrobial substance was responsible.

He was right. The substance he named magainin is found in the frog's skin. Magainin-like substances have been found in the human digestive system, which may explain why your cheek doesn't get infected when you accidentally bite it, despite the presence of all sorts of bacteria in your mouth. Other magainins shield the human brain.

Magainin is chemically able to break down the outer membrane of bacteria and other infectious invaders. In test-tube experiments (as well as in frogs), magainin has displayed its killing power against a whole spectrum of viruses, bacteria, fungi, and protozoa. Magainin is very active against *Acanthamoeba*, the microorganism associated with severe eye infections in contact-lens wearers. It's even being lab tested against human cancer cells.

True, there are a few infectious organisms that don't seem to be significantly affected by magainin. But the balance is currently in magainin's favor.

Scientifically speaking, magainin is a peptide, formed by a combination of amino acids. That means it can be reproduced synthetically at low cost and high efficiency. Dr. Zasloff has tested a synthetic magainin, and it seems to work as well as the natural peptide.

Synthesis of new magainins (over 400 so far) and development of practical applications for "magainin technology" are now handled by Magainin Sciences, Inc., Plymouth Township, Pennsylvania.

According to the company's medical director, Leonard Jacob, M.D., Ph.D., clinical trials to test efficacy and safety are currently being designed. Magainin products for human use (fighting infections in eyes and mouth, and severe burns) are expected to be on the market within several years.

Beating Cancer with Tobacco?

Smoking will never be good for your health, but in an ironic twist, the tobacco plant itself might someday become a genetic factory for cancer-fighting substances.

And this is not just some health-conscious scientist's idea of revenge. Tobacco has been the darling of plant geneticists for years because its cells are easy to invade. And once you invade a plant cell, you can sometimes put it to work making important substances that simply cannot be created in any other way. One of the easiest and safest methods of invading tobacco cells is to use a plant virus that attacks only tobacco. It's easy because the virus already knows how to invade the cell, and it can carry extra genetic material with it. It's safe because the basic reproductive material of the plant remains unchanged.

That means it won't pass on the virus-added genes and form a line of mutants.

The altered virus can carry genes that are programmed to make specific, useful proteins inside the tobacco cell. Once they're in, they turn the cell into a genetic factory. The theorized end result: Up to 40 percent of the dry weight of the tobacco leaf will consist of the desired protein.

There are a number of cancer-fighting proteins that could be made inexpensively by this method. Interleukin–2, a human immune system protein, is one of the more promising possibilities.

Melanin, the pigment protein that helps protect us against cancer-causing ultraviolet light, is another.

Right now the company that developed the gene/virus combination (Biosource Genetics Corp., Vacaville, California) is having success producing quantities of melanin in laboratory "bioreactors" containing tobacco cells. The company is seeking approval to market a melanin-based sunscreen for commercial use. Further testing of viruses on tobacco plants in the field is in the planning stages. A number of medically or industrially useful proteins could be selected for use for the first crop.

Electric Bandages for Pain?

Electric bandages sound like turn-of-the-century quackery. But this version has science by its side.

One of the better-known applications of electrical stimulation is something called TENS, which stands for transcutaneous electrical nerve stimulation. TENS is used to relieve chronic muscle pain. A small battery-powered TENS unit (hung on a belt or slipped in a pocket) delivers a very low electric charge to the muscle via two external electrodes. The theory behind TENS is that the electrical charge travels along the same nerve as the pain impulse, and they cancel each other out. It's like saying two wrongs make a right.

The electric bandage looks and works differently than TENS. It's merely an adhesive-backed fabric bandage impregnated with various metal particles. It has no external battery because you are the power source!

When the bandage makes contact with your skin, moisture from perspiration causes the metal particles to react with one another. The result is an extremely low level electrical charge that works directly on the muscle (not the nerves, as TENS does). The charge relieves pain by inducing muscle relaxation.

The electric charge generated by this bandage is many times lower than that given off by a TENS machine. The charge is so mild that the wearer can't even feel it. Yet studies show that the bandage does have a physically measurable effect: It causes muscles that have tightened in a spasm to relax.

So the bandage takes a few minutes to begin relieving pain, but it can be left on for several days. You can even get it wet! As many as 80 companies worldwide are investigating a similar electric bandage for use on open wounds to reduce healing time.

The American manufacturer (Medlec Corporation, Prior

Lake, Minnesota) of the muscle-relaxing bandage makes no such claim, but admits there may be good reasons for further study. They're seeking Food and Drug Administration (FDA) approval for marketing in this country.

A Cow Virus against Cancer?

A virus that makes cows sick may help keep some skin cancer patients well.

A mild bout of cowpox, a disease that affected both people and cows, was one of the occupational hazards of being a milkmaid. But cowpox provided immunity against smallpox, a related but much stronger disease that left facial scars. (In fact, years ago there was an expression "complexion like a milkmaid," which referred to clear, silky skin.) In the classic tale of scientific discovery, Dr. Edward Jenner noticed that milkmaids never got smallpox during epidemics. This led to the development of a smallpox vaccine from the cowpox virus.

Now the cowpox virus is part of a vaccine intended to halt cancer recurrence in people who have had surgery for malignant melanoma, the deadliest form of skin cancer.

There are many ongoing attempts to develop anticancer vaccines. But much of this work has been limited because each vaccine works on only one person—individuals have to be inoculated with their own cancer cells to boost the immune response. However, the experimental cowpox melanoma vaccine is intended to help a wide variety of people.

Researchers have combined four different strains of melanoma cells with the relatively harmless cowpox virus. The resultant vaccine induces the immune system to form antibodies against melanoma cells, reinforcing the response to the first cancer.

It's hoped that these antibodies will be capable of destroying any melanoma cells left in the body, and ambush any precancerous or normal cells that convert to full-blown cancer.

In preliminary clinical trials, the vaccine has successfully raised antibody levels in the blood of more than half of the test patients. "We're not yet sure if this will increase overall survival," says Eva Singletary, M.D., chief of the Melanoma Surgical Section at M. D. Anderson Cancer Center. But there seems to be some success in preventing the recurrence of melanoma. Equally as important, there seem to be few and very mild side effects to the vaccine, even at fairly high doses.

More definitive clinical trials have begun with more than 30 patients. Seven centers direct the trial: University of Texas M. D. Anderson Cancer Center (Houston); University of Florida (Gainesville); University of Alabama (Birmingham); Emory University (Atlanta); Duke University (Durham, North Carolina); Mount Sinai Medical Center (Miami Beach, Florida); and University of Colorado Cancer Center, Denver.

A Tree
vs. Ovarian Cancer?

A drug derived from the Western yew tree is a possible ally for women with ovarian cancer, even though the tree is itself an endangered species. Ovarian cancer is rare but deadly. When diagnosed at an advanced stage, the five-year survival rate is about 23 percent. The odds are significantly better (85 percent) if the cancer is caught early. But ovarian is a "silent" cancer. It often has few obvious symptoms in its early stages. The most common treatment for ovarian cancer is surgery, followed by a course of chemotherapy with a drug called cis-platinum.

But for those women who don't respond to this treatment for ovarian cancer, there may be hope in the form of Taxol, a new drug made from the bark of the Western yew tree.

Taxol, like many other anticancer drugs, inhibits the reproduction of cells. Any type of cell that reproduces rapidly—like a cancer cell—takes the greatest beating. Clinical studies have shown Taxol to be quite powerful. It not only inhibits tumor growth, but it also has strong side effects. The most disturbing is that high doses of Taxol seem to slow down the heart.

But for women who've failed to respond to cis-platinum

treatment for ovarian cancer, Taxol may be worth the risk. More than 30 percent of these women are responding favorably to Taxol. "We can't say any of these women have been cured yet," says George C. Lewis, Jr., M.D., director of gynecologic oncology at Jefferson Medical College in Philadelphia. "But their continued survival is an extremely promising sign."

And what of the endangered Western yew? There are two bits of good news: First, conservation efforts have begun to save the trees, and new ones are being planted. Second, the bark and leaves of a European yew tree produce a substance that seems to be similar to Taxol. The European yew is markedly more common, and if the drug can be made strictly from the leaves, entire trees won't be destroyed.

Taxol is now in stage II clinical trials at the cancer centers that participate in the National Cancer Institute's Gynecologic Oncology Group.

Saving Faces with Sea Coral?

The "catch of the day" in certain bone-replacement procedures is heat-toughened sea coral, which seems to work better than bone itself in some cases.

Certain types of sea coral are very similar to bone in pore structure. But the calcium carbonate of most coral would be quickly broken down if implanted in its natural state. So the coral must be combined with phosphates and water to convert it to hydroxyapatite (*hi-DROKS-ee-AP-puh-tite*), a calcium phosphate that is the major component of bone.

In a regular bone graft, a piece of bone is taken from a donor site on the patient, usually a section of rib or pelvis. Bone is living tissue, so once its blood supply is interrupted, it begins to degenerate. At the implant site, a regular bone graft will shrink, sometimes to a very noticeable degree. Cadaver-donated bone also has this shrinking problem.

But coral implants don't shrink. Their porous structure allows adjacent bone to grow into them, strengthening them over time. "I've had a very good success rate using coral implants for chin reconstruction," says Harvey M. Rosen, M.D., D.M.D., chief of plastic surgery at Pennsylvania Hospital and clinical associate professor of surgery at the University of Pennsylvania. "The implants are especially useful when the procedure is purely for cosmetic reasons, since there is only one operation (at the implant site) instead of two (implant and bone-harvesting sites)."

Coral is not perfect, though. The implants tend to be brittle, and some break while they're being attached.

But in Dr. Rosen's experience, no implant has shattered after it was secured in place. Coral has not been used in weight-bearing bones, however, because of its brittleness.

Right now, coral implants are approved by the FDA but are used on a limited basis because many surgeons are unfamiliar with them.

Chinese Cucumber vs. AIDS?

An extract of the Chinese cucumber plant is being tested to see if it can inhibit or even kill the AIDS virus in infected immune-system cells without harming normal cells.

A researcher at the Chinese University of Hong Kong discovered that trichosanthin, a protein extracted from the root of the Chinese cucumber plant, was able to cripple macrophages, a type of white blood cell. He brought this to the attention of Michael S. McGrath, M.D., director of the AIDS immunobiology research laboratory at San Francisco General Hospital. Dr. McGrath contacted a private company, Genelabs, and worked in conjunction with them to locate and purify the active ingredient in trichosanthin. They were successful. Now that active ingredient— called GLQ223—is being tested against the AIDS virus.

In laboratory studies, the San Francisco group discovered that GLQ223 seemed to block reproduction of the AIDS virus in T-cells, another component of the immune system.

While that's an important step in combating the virus, only a small percentage of T-cells become infected, and they usually die off soon afterward.

That's not so with macrophages. They can survive for a long time after becoming infected. Up to 7 percent of the macrophages in an AIDS patient's body appear to be infected with the virus. And those infected cells can infiltrate virtually every organ.

In test-tube experiments on the blood of eight people infected with the AIDS virus, GLQ223 seemed to kill infected macrophages while leaving uninfected cells alone. AZT, the only currently approved AIDS medication, does not kill infected cells—it merely inhibits replication of the virus. If GLQ223 is safe and effective in humans (it could turn out to be neither), it could theoretically destroy all the AIDS-virus–infected cells in a person's body.

Clinical trials to determine the safety and effectiveness of various injected doses of GLQ223 have begun at the University of California, San Francisco, and San Francisco General Hospital.

Experts caution that without medical supervision, using substances derived from the Chinese cucumber—sometimes called "compound Q"—can be extremely dangerous.

Cancer Drugs from Breasts?

A substance produced in the human breast to inhibit hormone-stimulated cell growth is being eyed as a future breast cancer treatment.

The substance is called mammastatin, a protein made by human mammary cells. If scientists can figure out exactly how mammastatin production is triggered, in theory they may be able to make breast cancer cells switch themselves off.

When a cell becomes cancerous, it grows and divides uncontrollably. In effect, the growth-inducing hormones in the cell overpower the growth-regulating hormones. According to laboratory tests at the University of Michigan Cancer Center, it seems that a relatively small counterdose of mammastatin may inhibit this uncontrolled cell growth. One application of mammastatin inhibited cell reproduction by 21 to 61 percent! (The tests were done in lab containers, not in humans.) Mammastatin was effective only against cancer cells taken from the breast—it didn't have much of an effect against cancer cells taken from other parts of the body.

Another curious quirk: Mammastatin may be useful in predicting who's at greatest risk of breast cancer.

All women have mammastatin in their bodies. A certain amount of it circulates through the bloodstream. Some women have a lot; some, only a little. The Michigan researchers are trying to see if there's a link between these blood levels and the development of cancer.

Right now, all work with the recently discovered mammastatin is in the experimental stage. Perhaps scientific curiosity will uncover mammastatin-like substances in other cells that can "turn off" cancer—leading to a whole host of medical miracles for the most perplexing of diseases.

CHAPTER 6

Ironing Out
Erratic Heartbeats

Arrhythmias are the heart disease most cardiologists know the least about, but the field of electrophysiology is changing that.

In early September 1982, Samuel W. suffered an unexpected and very serious heart attack. But as bad and incomprehensible as his heart attack was, what followed was numbing.

Because of Samuel's age and the advanced disease discovered in his heart, his cardiologists ruled out cardiac bypass surgery, feeling that it would be a life-threatening gamble with few potential rewards. Rather, the physicians prescribed a heart-stabilizing drug to at least thwart Samuel's uncomfortable, but mild, erratic heartbeats—a symptom that emerged as a by-product of his heart attack.

Within weeks, however, Samuel had a marked reaction to the medication in the form of a severe rash that covered his body, and he was taken off it. No new medication was prescribed. But without any drugs to stabilize his heart rhythm, for the next 2½ years, he suffered a series of discomforting incidents. Some were benign—merely dull pains that literally came and went in a matter of seconds;

others were breathtaking—dizzying episodes that brought him to the brink of passing out before he just as suddenly recovered.

Then, on a hot, humid afternoon in July 1985, while Samuel's children and their families were visiting him and his wife, something very weird happened. He was in mid-conversation when, without warning, his heart pitched forward into overdrive and in seconds was pounding at a rate more than three times its normal speed. At one point it was racing at 200 beats per minute.

"I felt as if something otherworldly had taken control of my body and pushed my heart almost to the point of bursting," he says. Frightened and sweating profusely, he ran into the bathroom to splash water on his face, to calm the turmoil somehow. But before he stepped out of the bathroom, he blacked out and fell to the floor.

Miraculously, Samuel lived through his cardiac electrical storm. And once he was stabilized at the hospital, it took only the briefest of examinations for his physicians to identify what the latest manifestation of Samuel's cardiac disease was all about: His superrapid pulse, worse than any erratic heartbeat he had suffered before, had been triggered by what became a broadly based electrical malfunction in his heart known as a ventricular arrhythmia.

Dangerously Offbeat

Samuel's case is not at all atypical. Ventricular arrhythmias are the most common of all heart conditions. They play a role in over 400,000 sudden deaths each year in this country alone, more than two-thirds of all deaths linked to heart disease. (Interesting enough, the arrhythmias that people are most aware of are not ventricular. These arrhythmias—called sinus tachycardia and atrial tachycardia—are usually completely harmless.) Sadly, arrhythmias are also the heart disease that most cardiologists know the least about. Many believe that there is little that can be done to avert an episode like Samuel's. But, now, thanks to a handful of pioneering scientists, dramatic new diagnostic techniques and treatments may offer arrhythmia patients a life that is more normal—free of the constant fear of an impending cardiac catastrophe.

The Heart of the Matter

The heart, it turns out, is not merely muscles and blood; rather it is a hot-wired organ, dependent on steady and unfailing electrical impulses to perform as an efficient pump.

In ventricular tachycardia, the heart beats far too fast and does not have enough time to fill its chambers with incoming blood before pumping. The heart ceases to deliver blood effectively to the lungs or throughout the body, and the result is vastly diminished blood pressure or a loss of consciousness.

Ventricular tachycardia may be followed by a second electrical disturbance known as ventricular fibrillation. Ventricular fibrillation is a chaotic rhythm in which the pumping chambers of the heart, the ventricles, cease to pump blood altogether. The result, unless treated within seconds, is fatal.

Ventricular tachycardia and fibrillation are deadly time bombs set randomly and silently. They are isolated electrical catastrophes that, in those prone to electrical malfunctions of the heart, may occur once a month, once a year, or never in the most fortunate. Yet, in those of us wired to explode, they are often undetectable. Moreover, some ventricular arrhythmias operate so quietly until they attack with a full frontal assault that for many, death—sudden and often untimely—caused by an arrhythmia is the first and only manifestation of a heart problem that they will ever have.

Contributing Factors

The most common cause of these life-threatening ventricular arrhythmias is any form of damage to the heart muscle, such as ischemia (a dangerous reduction in the blood supply to the heart) or atherosclerosis (a narrowing or blockage of coronary arteries); a cardiac scar, which occurs after a heart attack and after a long interruption of blood flow; and hypertrophy (enlargement) of cardiac cells, which often is caused by such conditions as severe high blood pressure. In each of these cases, when the heart muscle is compromised, its electrical system is disturbed in the process.

What's more, it appears, our habits and emotions may be even deadlier than our diseases. For instance, there has been a frightening upturn recently in the number of sudden cardiac deaths due to arrhythmia among young people and those who ply the upwardly mobile fast track, because of the increasing use of so-called recreational drugs like cocaine and, to a lesser extent, marijuana.

Traditional Treatment

The traditional method of treating life-threatening arrhythmias is to prescribe drugs. But studies have shown that up to 40 percent of arrhythmia patients treated this way will have another life-threatening cardiac electrical malfunction within one year.

But it's not only that drugs often fail to stem arrhythmias. Ironically, they sometimes actually increase the chance of tachycardia and fibrillation.

"If we have learned one thing in the last ten years," says Jeremy Ruskin, M.D., director of the Cardiac Arrhythmia Service at Massachusetts General Hospital in Boston, "it is that we cannot reach up on the shelf, pull down a bottle, hand it to a patient with tachycardia and say, 'Here take this and go home. It will work for you,' in the way that we can with penicillin or erythromycin for a streptococcal infection of the throat."

New, Nontraditional Solutions

Dr. Ruskin is one of a new generation of cardiologists—called cardiac electrophysiologists—attacking arrhythmias with nontraditional, inspired solutions. During a two-year period, 90 percent of the critically ill patients they've treated are free of life-threatening arrhythmias.

Advances in cardiac electrophysiology are occurring so

frequently now that researchers are building on each other's breakthroughs, constructing a pyramid of medical achievements that none would have thought possible just a decade ago.

As an example, clinical and laboratory investigators have produced computer-created, three-dimensional depictions of the stages and breakdowns in normal performance as a healthy heart deteriorates into an arrhythmic mass of uncadenced muscle.

And on an even more vital plateau that has immediate import for patients with arrhythmias, Michel Mirowski, M.D., of Baltimore's Sinai Hospital, has created a device called an automatic implantable cardioverter defibrillator (AICD). A 3-inch-wide piece of titanium that is embedded under a patient's skin near the abdomen and plugged into the heart with electrodes, the AICD continuously monitors the electrical activity of the ventricles. When the internal rhythm becomes dangerously fast, without prompting, the device delivers a countershock that normalizes the pulse beat. The one-year arrhythmia mortality rate of patients with arrhythmias who have had cardioverter defibrillators installed is a meager 2 percent.

One of the first to ambitiously research sudden cardiac death and the use of electrophysiological techniques in patients with ventricular tachycardia was the Dutch physician Hein Wellens, M.D. Dr. Wellens found that arrhythmias could frequently be reproduced and terminated in these patients using carefully timed electrical stimuli delivered to the ventricles through a catheter. A few years later, Mark Josephson, M.D., and his colleagues at the University of Pennsylvania, in Philadelphia, confirmed and expanded these observations and carried out pioneering research on the mechanisms of ventricular tachycardia.

Critical insights gained from their research into the mechanisms of ventricular arrhythmias—and the newfound ability to start and stop some forms of ventricular tachycardia in the controlled environment of a clinical laboratory—intrigued Dr. Ruskin at Massachusetts General in Boston.

Dr. Ruskin and his associate, Hasan Garan, M.D., began conducting similar studies on patients who had been successfully resuscitated from an episode of cardiac arrest. They identified 31 patients who had collapsed suddenly and unexpectedly of ventricular arrhythmias. Following resuscitation and recovery, these patients were temporarily in stable condition but were known to be at extremely high risk for another potentially fatal cardiac arrest.

The patients were observed in an intensive-care unit while their use of anti-arrhythmic drugs was discontinued for several days. Doctors then inserted a series of electrode catheters into veins in the thigh and arm. Monitored through a fluoroscope, the electrodes were positioned at several different sites within the heart. A variety of programmed electrical pulses was then delivered through the catheters to the heart in an attempt to provoke ventricular arrhythmias.

Ventricular arrhythmias were induced in 25 of the 31 patients. (Of the 6 other patients, 2 had ventricular arrhythmias that, ironically, could only be induced when they were taking anti-arrhythmic drugs; in the 4 additional cases, either no cardiac rhythm abnormalities were found on further testing or the patient had an atrial and not a ventricular arrhythmia.) The induced ventricular arrhythmias were quickly stopped with countershocks, returning the heart rhythm to normal in all patients.

This experiment and others like it occurring across the country at the same time were watersheds in both electrophysiology and cardiology. Cardiologists were finally face-to-face with the deadly ventricular arrhythmia on their terms. Because they could at last turn a ventricular arrhythmia on and off at will, they could now examine it as it occurred—the first step to understanding it and ultimately disabling it with drugs or other forms of therapy.

Most important, electrophysiologists could finally design clinical strategies to counter the fruitless methods previously used to treat patients who survived cardiac arrest. Heart disease is a complex condition but, in many cases, performing surgery on coronary arteries or on cardiac valves while ignoring the underlying arrhythmias is like seeing a patient with severe emphysema and a bloody nose, merely stopping the nosebleed, and pronouncing the patient cured. The other condition, the one that will probably be fatal before long, is left to continue to do its damage.

Tailoring the Treatment

The first clinical strategy that emerged from the ability to induce ventricular arrhythmias in the catheterization lab is a reworking of an old technique that had failed patients time after time: the random use of anti-arrhythmic drugs.

Now that ventricular arrhythmias can be started and stopped in the laboratory, electrophysiologists are able, with trial and error, to test the efficacy and safety of anti-arrhythmic drugs before sending a patient home with a bottle of pills. First, a drug—perhaps quinidine or procai-namide—is administered to the patient for several days. Second, electrical stimulation of the heart is repeated in an attempt to make the ventricular arrhythmia recur in the catheterization lab. If no sign of ventricular tachycardia or fibrillation appears, the drug is considered adequate. But if a ventricular arrhythmia ensues, alternative medications are assessed in the cath lab until an adequate drug regimen is found.

This trial-and-error procedure is significant. It breaks the vicious circle that a patient can suffer for years as drug after drug fails and a drastically diminished quality of life is a result of the side effects and the inefficacy of randomly prescribed combinations of toxic pharmaceuticals.

Too often—in at least one-third of all patients treated by electrophysiologists—drugs are still not the solution for cardiac arrhythmias. In those cases, options such as anti-arrhythmia surgery and the implantation of an automatic defibrillator to prevent or terminate the arrhythmia when it occurs are used.

"The treatment of cardiac arrhythmias at Massachusetts General and other centers that specialize in this problem is a very complicated one because of the large number of relatively new therapeutic options that have become available," adds Dr. Ruskin.

Fortunately, for Samuel W., his cousin, who lives in Boston, suggested that he be examined at Massachusetts General. To take a trip north was perhaps the best advice

Samuel received. Miraculously, one laboratory test and one operation later, Samuel was discharged from the hospital a much healthier man.

CHAPTER 7

A Guide
to High
Blood Pressure Drugs

By Marvin Moser, M.D.

The dozens of medications don't all produce the same results. Find out which one may be preferred in your situation.

A 46-year-old truck driver, W.S., first learned he had high blood pressure when his dentist took a routine reading. He saw his doctor, who confirmed that his pressure was 180/110. He was put on medication, which brought his pressure down to a near-normal level of 125/85.

At this point W.S. thought his hypertension was cured and he could stop taking the pills.

Six months later he was admitted to a hospital with heart failure. Fortunately, he survived and is now doing fine. But had he followed his doctor's instructions to keep taking his medication, W.S. could have averted this major complication of hypertension.

We now have abundant scientific evidence that reducing even slightly elevated high blood pressure lessens the risk of a heart attack or stroke, or kidney failure. Some people with mild to moderate hypertension can control their blood pressure with diet, exercise, and other behavioral approaches. But the majority still require some sort of medication to achieve and maintain normal readings.

Physicians disagree on when antihypertensive drug therapy should be started and what drugs should be used first. A report from the National High Blood Pressure Education Program stresses that the benefits of drug therapy outweigh any known risks to individuals with persistently elevated diastolic pressure (the bottom number in the blood pressure equation, representing the resting pressure) above 94 millimeters of mercury (mm Hg)—or above 90 in persons who smoke, have high blood cholesterol, or are otherwise at high risk for cardiovascular disease.

I am one of many physicians who recommend drug therapy for any patient whose diastolic blood pressure is consistently above 90 after a three- to six-month trial of diet and exercise. A number of extensive studies have shown that the risk of a fatal stroke or heart attack can be reduced by lowering blood pressure that is consistently above this level. I also believe that when the systolic blood pressure (the top number in the blood pressure equation, representing pumping pressure) is consistently higher than 140, it should be lowered by medicines if, of course, nondrug treatment hasn't worked.

Keep in mind, too, that just as some doctors neglect to treat high blood pressure adequately, others err in the opposite direction; they overtreat it. Unless your blood pressure is very high on the first visit—say, above 150/100—or you have other specific risk factors for heart disease, there is usually no need to start medication immediately. Instead, you should probably be told to restrict your salt intake, increase physical activity, and, if needed, stop smoking and begin to lose excess weight. You should return for a second checkup in about two or three months.

Types of Drugs

If blood pressure–lowering medications are necessary, the next step is to determine which drug (or drugs) will work best for you. Fortunately, today, we have dozens of different drugs to choose from. They fall into the following categories.

Diuretics. These drugs increase the excretion of sodium and water by the kidneys. They thereby reduce the volume of blood in the arteries and veins and consequently lower blood pressure. Also, loss of sodium in the blood vessel walls may help dilate them and thereby help lower blood pressure.

Thiazide diuretics are the most commonly used and are well tolerated by most patients. The so-called loop diuretics usually are reserved for patients whose blood pressure is not controlled with thiazide diuretics or who have kidney complications or heart failure. A third class is called the potassium-sparing diuretics. They are mostly used along with a thiazide or loop diuretic to help the body retain potassium while eliminating excessive sodium.

Diuretics alone lower blood pressure in about 40 to 50 percent of hypertensive persons. When used in combination with other drugs, their success rate rises.

Beta-blockers. These block the automatic responses of certain nerve receptors (beta-receptors). They prevent these receptors from signaling an increase in the heart rate during activity, for example. And they reduce the amount of blood pumped with each beat, which helps lower blood pressure.

About 80 to 85 percent of patients who are given a diuretic plus a beta-blocker have their pressures lowered to normal.

Angiotensin converting enzyme (ACE) inhibitors. These are drugs that prevent the production of a powerful blood vessel constrictor, angiotensin II. Angiotensin II also causes retention of salt and water.

Newcomers in the hypertension field, the ACE inhibitors are very effective and have been associated with relatively few side effects. If, however, a person's blood pressure is well controlled with another drug without undue side effects, there is no reason to change to one of these newer agents.

Calcium channel blockers. These block the entry of calcium into blood vessel walls. As a result, blood vessels relax and dilate.

These drugs are effective as initial treatment in about 30 to 40 percent of patients, but they are no more effective (and perhaps even less so in some patient groups) than diuretics or beta-blockers.

Vasodilators. These drugs dilate arteries. This allows blood to flow more easily through the arteries; resistance is lowered, and blood pressure is reduced. These medicines are usually given along with a beta-blocker or other nerve inhibitor and a diuretic.

Alpha-blocking agents. These are drugs that block receptors on blood vessel walls (alpha-receptors) that, when stimulated, constrict the vessels. When they are blocked, dilation of the arteries results.

Since prazosin and terazosin (two common alpha-blocking agents) can cause fainting, care must be taken when use of these drugs is begun. Patients starting on either agent should be careful to avoid standing suddenly, since an abrupt change in position can cause a fall in blood pressure and result in dizziness or fainting.

I usually reserve alpha-blockers for patients who have not had their blood pressures adequately controlled with other agents. These drugs are particularly useful for individuals with persistently elevated diastolic blood pressures.

Peripheral adrenergic antagonists. These block the release of norepinephrine (adrenaline) in response to stress. The oldest drug in the category is reserpine, which is made from the roots of the rauwolfia plant of India. In fact, these drugs were used in some Eastern societies for years because of their calming, sedative effect.

The use of reserpine has decreased over the years, but I still continue to give it to selected patients, never as initial therapy but in combination with a diuretic. About 70 to 80 percent of patients respond with normal blood pressure.

Centrally acting drugs. These drugs dilate the peripheral arteries. They may lower heart rate to some degree but do not have a major effect on the amount of blood pumped out by the heart.

I rarely, if ever, use centrally acting drugs as initial treatment. They are usually given along with a diuretic if it has failed to lower blood pressure. Occasionally I use them as third or even fourth drugs in patients whose blood pressure is difficult to control.

Combination drugs of blood pressure–lowering medications are available. These can be used after an effective dosage of each drug has been achieved. For example, if blood pressure is well controlled after several months of treatment with 80 milligrams of a beta-blocker, such as propranolol, plus 25 milligrams per day of a diuretic, such as hydrochlorothiazide, the patient might appropriately be switched to a drug that provides a combination of these two drugs in a single pill.

Patients are rarely started on combination therapy because if side effects occur, it would be difficult to determine which agent is responsible. Also, it's possible that one agent alone would be sufficient to lower blood pressure. An exception might be for patients whose blood pressures are severely elevated.

Special Considerations

Usually, a patient is started on a low dose of one of the following: a thiazide diuretic, a beta-blocker, a calcium channel blocker, or an ACE inhibitor. If the initial prescription does not produce the desired results, the dosage is increased. If the desired blood pressure goal is not achieved, a small dose of one of the other drugs is added to the treatment. Sometimes a third or fourth drug is required.

Of course, choosing the right drug treatment for you is a very individualized process. Depending on your situation, certain drugs may be preferred. For example:

- If you are over age 60, diuretics and calcium channel blockers generally are more effective than beta-blockers. Avoid drugs causing depression (e.g., reserpine or some centrally acting drugs). Prazosin, terazosin, guanethidine, or guanadrel must be used with care; abnormally low blood pressure may result from their use.
- If you are young, a beta-blocker may be particularly useful, but exercise performance may be decreased in some individuals.
- If you are black, diuretics and calcium channel blockers are effective. Black patients do not respond as readily to

Occasional Reactions to Blood Pressure–Lowering Drugs

These are the most common side effects noted, but this does not mean they occur frequently. Actually they occur in only about 10 to 15 percent of patients taking the drugs listed. And they can be resolved. Talk to your physician.

Generic Names	Some Possible Side Effects
Diuretics Thiazide or thiazide-like drugs; indapamide; loop drugs—furosemide, bumetanide, ethacrynic acid	Weakness, muscle cramps, joint pains (gout), sexual dysfunction
Beta-blockers Propranolol, metoprolol, atenolol, acebutolol, nadolol, timolol, pindolol, labetolol (also an alpha-blocker)	Insomnia, nightmares, slow pulse, weakness, asthmatic attacks, cold hands and feet, dizziness, sexual dysfunction—varies with drugs
ACE inhibitors Captopril, enalapril, lisinopril	Skin rash, loss of taste, weakness, cough, palpitations, headache
Calcium channel blockers Nifedipine, verapamil, diltiazem, nicardipine	Swelling of legs, dizziness, palpitations, headaches, flushes, constipation (with verapamil or diltiazem)
Miscellaneous Rauwolfia drugs	Stuffy nose, nightmares, depression
Methyldopa	Drowsiness, fatigue, depression, impotence, fever
Hydralazine	Headaches, rapid heartbeat, joint pains

(continued)

Occasional Reactions to Blood Pressure-Lowering Drugs—Continued

Generic Names	Some Possible Side Effects
Minoxidil	Headaches, rapid heartbeat, excessive hair growth, fluid retention
Guanethidine, guanadrel	A form of impotence, dizziness, diarrhea
Clonidine, guanabenz	Dry mouth, drowsiness, fatigue
Prazosin, terazosin	Faintness after first few doses, palpitations

NOTE: Not all available drugs or all possible side effects are included in this list.

ACE inhibitors as white patients, unless treatment also includes a diuretic.

- If you are pregnant, methyldopa, hydralazine, and beta-blockers appear to be safe and effective. Many obstetricians are reluctant to use diuretics.
- If you have heart failure, diuretics and ACE inhibitors may be especially effective. Vasodilators and alpha-blockers also have beneficial effects.
- If you have kidney failure, loop diuretics (furosemide or bumetanide) and vasodilators (especially minoxidil) are particularly useful. Potassium-sparing diuretics and guanethidine should be used with caution.
- If you have angina pectoris, beta-blockers or calcium channel blockers are especially useful alone or with a diuretic (with a potassium-sparing component). Avoid drugs that cause rapid heartbeat (vasodilators) unless given with a beta-blocker.
- If you have had a heart attack, beta-blockers are the drugs of choice. They protect against a second heart attack. If blood pressure is not controlled, add a diuretic/potassium-sparing combination.
- If you have diabetes, ACE inhibitors may have specific

beneficial effects on your kidneys. Use of diuretics or beta-blockers may adversely affect blood glucose levels, but this is not common or important in most instances. Alpha-blockers are usually well tolerated. Beta-blockers may mask symptoms of insulin shock. Potassium-sparing diuretics should be used with caution.

- If you have had a stroke or ministroke, probably you should avoid (or use with great care) drugs that may cause a decrease in standing blood pressure (e.g., alpha-blockers, such as prazosin or drugs like guanethidine).
- If you have asthma or chronic lung disease (emphysema, or other), calcium channel blockers may protect against asthma that comes on after exercise. ACE inhibitors and diuretics are okay. Avoid beta-blockers.
- If you have Raynaud's disease (white fingers or toes in cold weather), nifedipine, methyldopa, reserpine, diuretics, prazosin, and guanethidine may be used, but avoid beta-blockers.
- If you experience episodes of severe rapid heartbeats, a beta-blocker or a calcium channel blocker, such as verapamil, may be the drug of choice. If blood pressure is not controlled, add a diuretic and make certain blood potassium levels do not decrease.
- If your heart rate is slower than 50 beats per minute, avoid beta-blockers, verapamil, and diltiazem.
- If you have elevated cholesterol levels, have blood chemistries checked periodically if you are taking beta-blockers or diuretics.
- If you have gout, diuretics may precipitate an acute attack in predisposed patients and in those with kidney failure.
- If there is a history of depression, ACE inhibitors, diuretics, vasodilators, alpha-blockers, and guanethidine do not worsen or precipitate depression. Reserpine should be avoided. Centrally acting drugs (like methyldopa and clonidine) and beta-blockers may cause or exacerbate depression.
- If there is sexual dysfunction, vasodilators, alpha-blockers, ACE inhibitors, and calcium inhibitors may not affect sexual function as much as other antihypertensive drugs do.

- If you have osteoporosis (thinning of the bones), diuretics (except loop diuretics) may help preserve bone structure.
- If you have migraine headaches, beta-blockers and calcium channel blockers may be helpful.

Final Notes

Don't hesitate to ask your doctor questions. You should have a clear understanding of what you might expect from medications and be alert to possible side effects.

Medications to lower blood pressure are like any other drugs; there is always a certain risk of adverse reactions or undesired side effects (see "Occasional Reactions to Blood Pressure-Lowering Drugs" on page 73). However, the actual incidence of problems has, in my experience, been greatly exaggerated. Many patients come to me fully expecting that their lives will change once they go on medication. Most are pleasantly surprised to find that the medications are very well tolerated and when problems do occur, they usually can be remedied by alteration of the dosage or a switching of drugs.

Sometimes I run across an unusual side effect that is not generally associated with a medication. For example, I was seeing a patient who developed a dry, hacking cough. He was taking an ACE inhibitor (captopril). I asked when he had first noticed his coughing and, checking back in his records, I noted that it coincided with his starting the drug. I decided to substitute another drug, and sure enough the cough disappeared.

Be sure to contact your doctor if any unusual symptoms appear. In any event, you should not stop taking the medication on your own, nor in most cases should you try to adjust your own dosage.

CHAPTER 8

Raising Cholesterol?

By George L. Blackburn, M.D., Ph.D.

While high cholesterol is 20 times more common, low cholesterol causes big problems for some people.

"Mine's 250, so my doctor says I need to get it down."

"Well, I was just tested at 200. I'm very pleased."

If you're among health-conscious people, you're likely to hear a conversation like this. The numbers they're discussing, of course, are measurements of cholesterol.

Most Americans know by now that a high blood-cholesterol count is a health gamble. Anything over 200 can lead to clogged arteries and increased risk of cardiovascular disease, including heart attack and stroke. That's why many of us are cutting back on cholesterol and saturated fats and consuming more soluble fiber like oat bran, pectin, and guar gum (which may lower cholesterol).

A lot of people, though, are boasting of ultralow cholesterol numbers—of, say, 160 or lower. Is there such a thing as cholesterol levels that are too low?

The scientific consensus is that, for the majority of Americans, very low blood cholesterol (a reading below 160) is not a health risk. Research, however, does suggest that there might be a few people with certain health problems who should watch for cholesterol that's very low and who might actually need to raise it.

The Stroke Connection

Cholesterol itself isn't evil. In fact, it's essential for healthy living. The body produces cholesterol, and it's believed to be a critical factor in keeping vessel walls strong.

Too much cholesterol, however, can lead to strokes and other cardiovascular problems. Many people who suffer strokes—particularly the kind related to a blood clot in the brain or neck, called "cerebral thrombosis"—have blood cholesterol that's too high.

But there's another kind of stroke, a bleeding or "hemor-rhagic" stroke. It's not caused by a clot. Instead, blood vessels in the brain that might have a flaw or genetic weakness "blow out" and bleed. Bleeding strokes are far more likely to occur among people who have high blood pressure. This is the type of stroke that researchers have speculated might be associated with ultralow cholesterol because of the role cholesterol plays in the strengthening of blood vessels.

Support for this theory appeared in an important study published in the *New England Journal of Medicine*. It was an analysis of health data on 350,977 men, age 35 to 57. University of Minnesota researchers who analyzed the data found that men who had very high cholesterol were indeed at increased risk for strokes related to blood clots. And those with very low blood cholesterol were at three times greater risk for bleeding strokes than men with higher cholesterol. But the higher risk of death from bleed-ing strokes was limited to men who had both very low blood cholesterol (below 160) and high blood pressure (diastolic pressure, the second number, greater than or equal to 90). Men with high blood pressure are at greater risk for stroke to begin with, and the ultralow cholesterol apparently amplified the effect.

Keep in mind also that men who have both high blood pressure and very low cholesterol are also rare.

If You're Concerned

If you're a middle-aged man, and if your total cholesterol is below 160, you might want to ask your doctor to check whether you're one of the rare individuals for whom this could pose a problem.

And if you are that rare man at risk, you may in fact need to consume a little more saturated fat and cholesterol than current recommended levels. There simply isn't any evidence about what effect low cholesterol and high blood pressure might have on women or younger people. It's likely, however, that their risk is much lower.

Low Cholesterol and Immunity

There's one other subgroup of the population among whom low cholesterol should be a concern. In elderly men, ultralow cholesterol may be a marker for reduced immune function. Studies at Veterans Administration nursing homes have found that men with very low blood cholesterol are more susceptible to opportunistic infections. It's likely that both their cholesterol and their immune function are so low because they don't have much of an appetite and aren't eating a proper diet.

These people should be examined thoroughly by a physician and, depending on the findings, should possibly be put on a higher-fat diet.

For every American whose low cholesterol creates a health risk, I would venture to guess that 20 to 30 Americans have cholesterol that's too high. That's why everyone should get their cholesterol tested, including men, women, and children.

If you are a healthy adult, with no personal or family history of hypertension or cardiovascular disease and good health habits, then your cholesterol should ideally be no higher than 200. At 200, you have half the normal risk for heart disease.

If you do have a personal or family history of hypertension or cardiovascular disease, smoke, are overweight or sedentary, you need to be even more attentive to your cholesterol. Your cholesterol should be no higher than 200, and you may benefit by getting it a little lower, to about 180. Again, less than 180 is not dangerous for most people, but there's no physiological benefit from going lower. Don't strive for ultralow numbers unless you are under a special medical treatment.

Some people may be able to lower their high cholesterol significantly through diet or other lifestyle changes in only a month. (Others, however, may require drugs to get their cholesterol down.) At any rate, for every one-point drop in cholesterol, you can get a 2 percent drop in cardiovascular risk.

CHAPTER 9

The Diet
That Polishes
Arteries Clean

Dr. Dean Ornish's ground-breaking research suggests that to reverse heart disease, you may have to go beyond the American Heart Association's recommendations.

It's a handsome group, the 30 men and women gathering in a meeting room on the San Francisco waterfront this Tuesday evening. Most look fit and slender, and they chatter exuberantly as they come in from a brisk walk in the sunset shadow of the Golden Gate Bridge.

Heart disease is the last thing you'd think of if you met these people anywhere else, but they're here as participants in Dr. Dean Ornish's famous heart disease–reversal program. Bob Finnell, 53, with flashing dark eyes and erect posture, cuts a trim figure in his white running suit. "You should have seen me before I lost the 40 pounds," he laughs. He credits his weight loss to the program's vegetarian diet, and his officer's bearing to the yoga he's learned here. More important, blockages in six of his eight blocked heart arteries have diminished since he began the regimen.

At 75, Werner Hebenstreit is the oldest, but he neither looks nor moves his age—he's the group's fastest walker. Four years ago, his angina slowed him down so much that he couldn't make it across a city street before the light flashed to "Don't Walk." Now he and his wife, Eva, enjoy 6-hour mountain hikes. Blood flow to his heart has increased by more than 36 percent. "Sometimes I don't believe it myself!" he says. As the evening goes on, there will be more testimonials like these. This diverse assortment of heart patients—businesspeople, a minister, an engineer, and a contractor—didn't improve their health through cholesterol-lowering medication or bypass surgery.

Instead, they (and often their spouses) undertook a completely new way of life, including moderate exercise, a very low fat vegetarian diet, yoga, and other stress-reduction practices, along with biweekly group therapy.

Their new lifestyle was prescribed by Dean Ornish, M.D., an assistant clinical professor of medicine at the University of California, San Francisco, and at Pacific Presbyterian Medical Center and author of *Dr. Dean Ornish's Program for Reversing Heart Disease.*

With these patients as evidence, Dr. Ornish's research suggests that diet and behavior changes can significantly reverse coronary blockages in just one year. His work is helping to change the way we think about heart disease. Just a few years ago, many authorities doubted whether blockages could be systematically reversed at all. But more recently, studies have shown that atherosclerosis (blocked arteries leading to the heart) can be diminished using medication.

"Dr. Ornish's work is very significant because he has achieved with diet and relaxation the same kinds of results other researchers have achieved with powerful cholesterol-lowering drugs," says William Castelli, M.D., medical director of the Framingham Heart Study. "But the measures he uses are nontoxic, and you can do them forever."

The catch: Reversing heart disease requires major lifestyle changes, not the least of which involves dropping total fat intake to a meager 10 percent of calories. That's why some physicians wonder about the practicality of the plan. "For those who do it, it works," comments Claude Lenfant, M.D., director of the National Heart, Lung and Blood Institute. "But there is a question about whether the public will accept this kind of regimen; I understand it's pretty tough."

Yet the participants we met insisted that adapting the new health habits wasn't so tough. What's more, they felt and looked so much better so quickly that the sacrifices were worth it. Bob Finnell jokes to a visitor, "As time has gone on, some of the visitors to our program look like the heart patients, and we look like potential astronauts."

It's true.

Understanding Ornish

To understand the Ornish program, you have to understand a little bit about Dean Ornish himself. He's young, but at 36, he's already had nearly two decades of experience with the lifestyle he recommends. In college, he was a stressed-out premed student, so nervous that he found himself afraid of failing a crucial organic chemistry class. He realized that he needed to change his life dramatically. So he took up yoga, meditation, and a vegetarian diet. "I had a lot more energy, I could think better, I felt better." He went on to graduate as class valedictorian.

In medical school at Baylor College of Medicine, in Houston, he became interested in whether the same lifestyle could benefit people with heart disease. Different studies had indicated that, for example, stress raises cholesterol; that meditation lowers blood pressure (at least temporarily); that high-strung, hard-driving behavior might harm the heart; and that vegetarian diets are associated with low risk of heart disease. But no one had put all the lifestyle factors together into one program.

So he did it, first as a medical student and then during a residency at the Harvard-affiliated Massachusetts General Hospital, in Boston. There he conducted small studies that suggested heart patients felt better and had improved heart function and blood flow when they kept to a vegetarian diet; did moderate exercise; and practiced yoga, meditation, and other stress-reduction techniques. He based his first book, *Stress, Diet, and Your Heart*, on this research.

In 1985, Dr. Ornish began recruiting people for a larger study that would use the newest technology to show the precise effects of the regimen on the heart. He located people with high degrees of atherosclerosis who had either refused, or who for medical reasons could not undergo, coronary bypass to open their blockages. Many had survived one or more heart attacks.

The patients—43 men and 5 women—were divided into two groups. The "treatment" group was instructed to go on a strict vegetarian diet deriving fewer than 10 percent of calories from fat. They were to stop smoking, do an hour of yoga and meditation daily, and exercise moderately (which usually meant walking) for at least 1 hour, three days a week, or 30 minutes every day. The members of the treatment group also made a commitment to attend an introductory week-long retreat and to meet twice a week, for four hours of group activities. During these meetings, they'd walk, participate in stress-management workshops, eat dinner, and engage in group therapy sessions led by Dr. Ornish. The program provided unlimited lunches and dinners to take home.

Meanwhile, the control group was advised to follow the standard AHA lifestyle prescription for heart health. That is, reduce their fat intake to under 30 percent of calories, stop smoking and exercise moderately. None of the patients in the treatment group used cholesterol-lowering drugs, although some people in the control group did.

The patients in both groups were queried regarding their diet, exercise, and stress-management practices at six-month intervals. (Few people in either group smoked.) Their progress was assessed annually, using quantitative angiography (an x-ray movie of the heart's arteries), and ultrasophisticated positron emission tomography (PET) scanning, which accurately shows blood flow through the heart.

As of November 1989, all the participants had completed one year of the program (and some had followed it for as long as four years). The one-year results, which Dr. Ornish announced at the American Heart Association meeting in New Orleans in the fall of 1989, made banner headlines nationwide. There were usable data on 41 of the 48 patients (22 in the treatment group and 19 in the control group).

In the treatment group, 82 percent had some reversal of coronary blockages. One got significantly worse "and he didn't follow the program very well," says Dr. Ornish. Three stayed about the same.

The blockage reductions—on the order of 5 percent—were small but significant, Dr. Ornish explains, because even small changes in blockages can have an enormous effect on the amount of blood the heart receives. (A 5 percent regression can mean a 100 percent improvement in blood flow—and, in some cases, even more.) "As a result, people began to feel better very quickly," says Dr. Ornish.

In the control group, however, the results were much less dramatic. While those who adhered to the AHA program fared better than those who didn't, they did not experience the striking reversals seen in the treatment group. At best, the men's disease appeared to progress at a slower rate.

In men, at least, these results suggest that to reverse heart disease you may have to go beyond the AHA recommendations, says Dr. Ornish. (For some reason, all the women—even those in the control group—showed some reversal in heart disease. But Dr. Ornish cautions that it's too early to draw conclusions since only five women participated in the study.)

Another interesting result: The more severe the disease, the more dramatic the improvement on Dr. Ornish's program. The patient with the worst heart disease, Bob Finnell, enjoyed the most clearing of his arteries. He was also among the most compliant.

And the better that people followed the program, the more reversal they had, Dr. Ornish notes.

All this should come as good news to people with atherosclerosis. "It's a program that worked for almost everyone in our study who followed it," says Dr. Ornish. "Apparently, it's never too late to begin making lifestyle changes. And the more lifestyle changes you make, the more improvement you're likely to show."

But how do you motivate people to change completely what they eat, how they spend their leisure, even how they think? They may be Californians, but most of the Ornish patients and their spouses (who were encouraged to participate) cheerfully admit that stuff like yoga and meditation wasn't on their agenda. "I never thought I'd be doing this," says Joe Cecena, 61, a retired government executive who'd suffered two heart attacks. "I thought yoga was strictly for females. I thought it was their exercise, it wasn't for me. Running or waterskiing or something like that was for me. Now, I don't feel right if I don't do my yoga and meditation every day." What happened to change their minds?

Opening Up

Dr. Ornish believes that there's a psychological component to heart disease. He's observed that heart patients often feel isolated and inadequate—"a sense of not having enough or being enough." In some people, these feelings of inadequacy lead to hostility, he says. He points out that the latest research on Type-A behavior suggests that hostility may be the most poisonous trait for the heart.

That's why group therapy, in which the members talk about their frustrations and learn to listen and open up to others, is central to the program. "One of the real values of the group is you can show parts of yourself that you think are going to cause you to be rejected, and you find you're accepted," says Dr. Ornish. "Then real intimacy can happen. And where there's intimacy there's healing, because you relieve some of the chronic stress and isolation that comes from having to hide who you really are."

Werner Hebenstreit says that opening up to the group changed his personality and his marriage and helped him deal with anger and stress.

His first heart attack came at 65, and his second, six years later. Yet both his diet and his exercise were exemplary: He was a vegetarian and an active outdoorsman leading Sierra Club expeditions. But his life had always been stressful. "I always felt I had to earn a lot of money.

"I was a typical Type-A personality: ambitious, time conscious, very serious, easily on the defensive. I had a short fuse, as they say.

"I was always a loner," he adds. "If I did join groups, I had to run them. In the Sierra Club, I always had to be the leader. People did things the way I wanted or there was trouble."

He was able to stay active after his first heart attack, but the second, at 71, left him feeling like an invalid. Even though he could still work, "I did everything in slow motion. I took 14 tablets of all different colors every day, with all the blasted side effects. I was mad at the world, and mad at myself, too."

Communications with his wife broke down. "I was short tempered when I came home. I didn't want to be bothered with her questions. 'Don't ask me!' I'd yell at her."

When Dr. Ornish telephoned to invite him to apply for the program, Hebenstreit's wife answered the phone—but Hebenstreit refused to take the call. "I said, 'Dammit, tell him I don't want to talk to doctors! I've had enough of doctors!' " But he finally agreed to meet Dr. Ornish, and in short order volunteered for the program.

"It was the first positive thing that came along," Eva Hebenstreit recalls. "This was the glimmer of hope that you grab for."

How soon did he start to feel better? "Perhaps it's wishful thinking, but I felt different after the week-long retreat," Hebenstreit says. "My cholesterol even went down a little in that time." His angina soon vanished. He didn't need his rainbow of pills, either, "except for a baby aspirin every other day." After one year, blood flow to his heart improved by 20 percent. His cholesterol dropped from a preprogram high of 305 to its current 135. "Incredible? Yes, most doctors don't even believe me, but it's documented," he says. Today, he has no physical restrictions at all—and he and his wife spent their last vacation hiking in the Grand Teton mountains.

The vegetarian diet wasn't much different from what he ate before (he had to cut out cheese and fish). But what was really new for Hebenstreit was a better way of relating to people and dealing with frustrations, taught by psychologists. "I learned to loosen up and talk about my feelings, which wasn't easy for me. I learned not to take offense easily." After four years of meeting twice a week, he says, "The group is my extended family."

He also developed a trick for coping with frustrations; he'd write down every negative thought on a pad that he carried with him. "On good days there would be 23 entries."

Identifying the negative thoughts helped him learn to dismiss them. "Now, when I'm frustrated, I start to laugh. I was a typical Type A when I came to the program. Now I'm a C-minus type. I'm a lot more easygoing."

Best of all is the improvement in his marriage. "Now we're partners," he says. His wife smiles at him. "I confirm," she says.

Learning to Love Yoga

What's nearly as striking as the fitness of the participants is their grace as they go about their 70-minute yoga routine, including the 12 postures of the sun salutation. While visitors totter, the group members move smoothly, unswayed even by the tenuous angle position: hands and toes on the floor, buttocks aloft.

It's rare to find a cardiac rehabilitation program that teaches yoga. Yet, interestingly, Dr. Ornish's data show that the amount of time spent doing yoga was correlated with reductions in coronary blockages just as changes in diet or exercise were.

The slow stretching and breathing techniques relax muscles, says Dr. Ornish, and promote feelings of peace. Yoga taught in his program ranges from simple stretches, deep three-part breathing, and progressive muscle relaxation to more esoteric practices like alternate nostril breathing and chanting. Chanting produces a calming effect, just as singing does, Dr. Ornish says. "We show people how to adapt these practices to fit their own cultural and belief systems," he adds.

Yoga is Bob Finnell's favorite part of the program. A couple of times a week he takes an outside yoga class. That means he often does 90 minutes of yoga a day.

If today he is a "yogaholic," it has a lot to do with the fact that up until four years ago he was a workaholic. As the president of a $30-million-a-year nonprofit organization, he worked 12-hour days, ate two dinners a night if he was attending two evening functions, arrived at the last minute for airplanes, collected speeding tickets, lost his temper, and never, ever walked the 20 minutes it would take to get from his apartment to his office on foot. "I didn't even realize I was sedentary."

At 48, while hiking in Yosemite National Park, he collapsed—then stood up and walked 3 miles back to the car. A few weeks later, in a doctor's office, he discovered that he'd had a heart attack. Two of the three major arteries to his heart were completely blocked, and one was three-quarters blocked. His condition was very serious. "Three of four cardiologists looked at my heart and said, 'You need an immediate bypass or you'll be dead in six months,' " says Finnell.

But when he was told he had a 1 in 20 chance of not surviving the operation, he refused. Then he was recruited for the Ornish program. "That was over four years ago," he recalls proudly.

When he began the program, he focused mainly on the diet, doing only the minimum walking and half hour of yoga stretches.

"I was scared of exercise," he says. "At first, I couldn't touch my toes. I couldn't do any of the inverted yoga positions, like a shoulder stand or a headstand."

After six months, he began taking other yoga classes. And he noticed good things happening. For one thing, waking up felt different. "You have to understand, when I used to wake up in the morning, it was like opening an old creaky barn door. I would unhinge my elbows and knees, take a hot shower to loosen up, and in the old days, drink coffee to get going.

"But after I started doing more yoga, I started waking up refreshed, like I'd been up for 3 hours. My joints weren't creaky and my head was clear."

His posture had been poor. "I was hunched over a desk, a typewriter, a computer for 20 years, and I had these muscles in the front that were shortened, and in my back that were lengthened. Over time, yoga stretched my muscles."

Most important, says Finnell, "It gave me confidence in my body. It gave me a sense of control and a tool to do something about it."

While Finnell still has serious heart disease and cannot return to full-time work, he's very active. In addition to yoga, he walks for an hour (about 4 miles) a day, five days a week. He went to Africa for a two-month visit. The plaque buildup in six of his eight blocked arteries has diminished, significantly improving blood flow to his heart. "That's irrefutable. You can see the pictures. It also confirms the way I feel," he says.

There are other markers of progress, too. "My weight was in the 180s. Now it's in the 140s. My cholesterol is in the 110s and the 120s, down from 235 at the time of my heart attack. There's no question in my mind that if I'd only done the other parts of the program, I wouldn't be feeling as well as I do. Yoga made the difference for me."

Meditation for Transformation

Meditation may help reduce stress. But its benefits go deeper. "At the end of a meditation, you are feeling more peaceful, stronger, and happier," says Dr. Ornish.

Joe Cecena wasn't sure he'd be able to do it, but now he relies on the feeling of peace that meditation gives him to get through the stresses of his life.

If anyone needed stress relief, it was Cecena. His first heart attack hit in 1983, when he was 54. "I was working for the State of California, in the unemployment office, with 13 people under me. It was stress, stress, stress.

"Then my father-in-law passed away, and I had to take care of his financial affairs. Soon after that, my own father had a stroke. Finally, my daughter, who had a drug problem, took off and left us with two grandchildren to raise." Nonetheless, after a month of recovery, he returned to work. "The whole ball of wax started again. I did go on the American Heart Association diet, skinning chicken, eating fish. I lost some weight—not as much as I wanted—and I gained it back." He carried more than 230 pounds on his 5-foot, 11-inch frame.

In 1985, Cecena was stricken with another heart attack, then a third a few days later, in the hospital. "They told me that the blocked arteries were behind my heart and I couldn't have a bypass because I'd only have a 50–50 chance of surviving the operation. I couldn't walk any-where without pain."

His wife, Anita, remembers this as a terrifying time. "After they told us Joe couldn't have a bypass, I used to look at him when he was asleep, you know, to see if he was still breathing . . . if he was still alive."

Then, two years ago, Cecena was offered a place in the Ornish program. Today he is so enthusiastic about it that he apologizes for sounding like a preacher, but it's under-standable. "I lost 54 pounds in the first six months of the program. My cholesterol started at 244; now it's down to 172. Last year I found out my blockages are clearing out.

"Now, I'm very active, he adds."I walk 4 miles every morning. Oh, and I just finished painting the house, inside and out."

Visualization (a form of meditation), he says, has helped him enormously. The program's visualization and yoga instructor, Mary Dale Scheller, worked with him to find a focus (an image to concentrate on while visualizing), a focus that Cecena personally found calming and uplifting.

For him, the image that worked had to do with experi-encing himself enjoying his favorite recreation: snorkeling.

"I handle stress beautifully now with meditation and visualization. When I get pressure from the grandchil-dren—this one wants to use the telephone, the other wants to go somewhere, and I have my own things to do—I go into another room, sit on the floor in the cross-legged position, close my eyes and meditate on the motion of waves. I visualize myself underwater in Cancun, snorkel-ing, or looking at a lake or the ocean. When I get up I feel like a new man."

For his wife, Anita, the relief is immeasurable. "Now I have a lot of peace of mind because I know Joe can be healthy."

A New Way of Eating

"The first week I couldn't stand the food, and I lost about a pound a day," recalls Jim Keith, 60, a carpenter and kitchen remodeler, who ultimately lost 50 pounds on the program. "Then my taste buds started to change. I came to kind of enjoy it."

"If I could change my life, anyone could: I was a real meat-and-potatoes man," says Dwayne Butler, 54. He lost 80 pounds after a year on the program.

The list of prohibited foods on the Ornish regimen may appear daunting to some. Although calorie intake is unlimited, the food selection isn't. No more meat or fish. No nuts. No chocolate. No coffee.

But a meal prepared in accordance with the stringent guidelines can be delicious, satisfying—even exciting. Lunch might include a brown-rice-and-pea salad—the rice cooked in vegetable broth and seasoned with vinegar, mustard, and dill pickles. A scarlet cole slaw, made from red cabbage, with a tasty base of nonfat yogurt, mustard, wine vinegar, and oregano. A basket of dark German bread. "Potato spears" (thick wedges of potato, baked at 450°F for about 20 minutes, until they puff up golden) dipped in salsa. And finally, "banana ice," a dessert you can whip up on the spot (whirl a couple of cut-up, frozen bananas in the food processor with a dollop of yogurt, a splash of apple juice, and some nonsugared berry jam). The results are as creamy sweet as any premium ice cream.

Staying with the Program

Dr. Ornish refuses to say that any one aspect of the program is more effective than any other. "I believe that the lifestyle changes, like meditation and yoga, are as important as the dietary ones."

One of the key lessons of his experiment, he says, is that habits can change quickly and completely. "In some ways it's easier to make big changes than little ones. That's because if you make comprehensive changes, you begin to feel so much better so soon. We don't tell people, 'Do this because you'll live longer.' We say, 'Do this because you'll live better, you'll enjoy life more.'

"If a person is unwilling to give up their steak and cheeseburgers, then I'll prescribe the cholesterol-lowering drugs," adds Dr. Ornish. But there are problems with these drugs, he notes. First the expense—as much as $2,000 a year. Second, there's a risk of side effects, which can range from cataracts to liver damage. Surgical options, such as heart bypass or angioplasty, may be the best choice for some people but are becoming more controversial. Evidence shows that arteries often reclog within months of the procedures.

"The point to me is that it's much safer and more rational to reestablish heart health through lifestyle changes if possible," he says. "Yet doctors always tell me, 'Your program is so radical!' Isn't it ironic that it's considered radical to exercise, relax, and eat a heart-healthy diet and conservative to take potent drugs?

"Cardiovascular disease kills more people than any other disease in America, more than all other diseases combined. Yet, I'm convinced it can be prevented, and often it can be reversed. For people who already have heart disease, if they're willing to make these changes, they might never need a bypass, drugs, or angioplasty."

Farewell to Cappuccino

There's one more surprise in store for a visitor to the Ornish program. It's that many of the spouses stick to the regimen almost as religiously as the participants. They leave their job early on Tuesdays and Thursdays to be on the San Francisco waterfront at 5 P.M. sharp. They've said farewell to cappuccino and learned to love caffeine-free teas and grain beverages. They walk daily, they sit in meditation, stretch with yoga. Why?

"I feel healthy doing this," says Phyllis Cardozo, sitting on an exercise mat beside her husband, John, a heart patient. "I was never very athletic, but it feels good to take a walk after work. I love the yoga; my mom is all bent over, and I see the need to do it. Best of all, the group therapy has allowed us to go deeper into our feelings, and it's improved our relationship.

"I don't do this program just for John," she laughs. "I'm much too selfish. I do it for myself."

Just Try It for a Week

Interested in the Ornish program? "I say, maintain your skepticism, just try it for a week," says Dr. Ornish. If you have angina and you follow the program carefully, "after one week the pain will probably diminish. Even if you don't have heart disease at all, you'll feel noticeably better and have more energy after a week."

One note of caution: If you do have heart disease, check with your doctor before undertaking this program. If you don't have heart disease but want to cut your chances of developing it, you may be able to adopt a modified version of Dr. Ornish's program. A one-week test run should give you a good feel for the program and what it can do for you.

The best way to test the Ornish regimen for yourself is to consult his book, *Dr. Dean Ornish's Program for Reversing Heart Disease*. It provides a detailed description of all aspects of the program.

In the meantime, here are some different components you can try for seven days.

The Intensive Healing Diet

Participants in Dr. Dean Ornish's program swear by his diet—though they admit it takes some getting used to. After all, the diet, which helps bring about dramatic results, delivers only 10 percent of calories from fat. "It's the way most of the world eats that doesn't get heart disease," says Dr. Ornish. The average American diet packs about 40 percent fat.

To achieve this drastic fat reduction, Dr. Ornish favors a vegetarian diet: that is, no meat, poultry, fish, or cheese. In addition, he advises his program participants to go easy on high-fat vegetable foods. This means cutting out nuts, seeds, and, of course, vegetable oils.

Caffeinated coffee and teas are also on Dr. Ornish's forbidden foods list. Caffeine probably doesn't damage the heart or arteries, he explains, but it can trigger irregular heartbeats in some people and may promote stress by making people jittery. So, what foods are permissible on this program? Plenty, and plenty of them. Dr. Ornish says his people can eat as much as they want of the following: Grains and grain products (preferably whole grains) such as bread, cereal, rice, pasta, and tortillas; fresh or dried fruits; vegetables and greens; beans; sprouts; and egg whites. Tofu and tempeh, which are naturally high in fat, are permitted in moderation. He also allows up to 1 cup of skim milk or nonfat yogurt a day.

And while Dr. Ornish discourages drinking alcohol, his diet does permit 2 ounces a day.

Many processed and convenience foods meet the guidelines, if they have no added oil or egg yolks and only a minimum of sugar and salt. Seasonings like herbs, of course, are fine, and so are mustard, salsa, and ketchup.

In general, the diet does not restrict salt. But Dr. Ornish recommends that salt-sensitive people, whose blood pressure responds dramatically to sodium levels, be more cautious about avoiding it.

Is this diet for you? There's little debate over the heart-healthy benefits of a low-fat diet. The question is, how low do you need to go to get the maximum protective effect?

The American Heart Association recommends that all of us, men and women, reduce our fat intake to under 30 percent of calories. The National Research Council agrees but adds that "further reduction in fat intake may confer even greater health benefits." The Pritikin Longevity Centers have long reported the cholesterol-lowering and "feel-better" benefits of a very low fat diet similar to Dr. Ornish's.

If you're healthy, with no sign of heart disease, you may do well following a less restrictive prevention diet. By adding moderate amounts of fish, lean meats and poultry, and unsaturated vegetable oils to the Ornish plan, for example, you'll still keep fat within the American Heart Association guidelines.

On the other hand, if you do have heart disease or a propensity to it, you may want to consider going the extra mile—that is, following Dr. Dean Ornish's diet to the letter. Talk to your doctor first, however. And keep in mind that, because this diet restricts certain foods, you should take a multiple vitamin and mineral supplement to ensure you're meeting all your nutritional needs.

The cholesterol benchmark. The goal of any heart-healthy diet (whether preventive or restorative) is primarily to reduce elevated blood cholesterol. The American Heart Association recommends dietary changes for anyone whose cholesterol level exceeds 200. Dr. Ornish believes that a very low fat diet could benefit others, too. "A cholesterol level below 150 will put you at the lowest risk of developing atherosclerosis and will increase the likelihood of reversing heart disease," he says.

If, however, your cholesterol won't go below 150, despite following a strict diet, don't worry. "Several of the patients in our study followed the diet and lifestyle program virtually 100 percent and showed some measurable reversal of their coronary atherosclerosis even when their blood cholesterol levels remained elevated."

A delicious way to eat. Whether you plan to give the Ornish diet a whole-hearted try (or modify it somewhat to meet your needs), you'll be pleasantly surprised by the variety and flavor of his vegetarian cuisine. "We're trying to show that food can be tasty, attractive, and beautifully presented, as well as healthful," says Dr. Ornish.

Moderate Exercise

Dr. Ornish is a believer in moderate exercise. "The equivalent of walking a half hour to an hour a day, according to the latest research, causes the greatest reduction in mortality. And beyond that you really don't get much more benefit, but the risks may go up substantially, especially for someone with severe heart disease."

So for the week, make sure that you're walking for 20 to 30 minutes a day (if you're a beginning exerciser) at a pace that doesn't feel like a strain. (Eventually, you can build up to brisk walks of 30 to 60 minutes duration.)

Another reminder for heart patients: Check with your doctor before beginning any exercise program, even if it's just for a week.

Yoga

Yoga stretches are best learned in a class with an instructor. You might want to contact your local YM/YWCA or check the yellow pages for the nearest "Integral Yoga Institute," which is where Dr. Ornish learned yoga. As an option, read Dr. Ornish's book. It details yoga routines, including the 12 flowing poses of the sun salutation. You can read the directions into a tape recorder, and then play back the tape as you do them. Or ask your video store for an instructional yoga tape. Never do anything that feels uncomfortable. "When you stretch and you feel so good that your body goes 'aahh,' you're doing it exactly right," says Mary Dale Scheller, the Ornish Program yoga instructor.

One of the foundations of yoga is proper breathing. There is a simple technique called three-part breathing that you can start right away at home.

The initial step: Sit up straight in a chair, with your spine erect, shoulders back, and head centered. Exhale fully. On the next inhale, feel your abdomen expand. Exhale, feeling the abdomen pulling in toward the spine. Do that a few times until the expansion and contraction come naturally. Then bring breathing back to normal and relax.

The next learning step: Exhale fully. Continue inhaling deeply, with the abdomen expanding, and the rib cage muscles expanding outward. When you exhale, feel the rib cage muscles contract and the abdomen pull in. Do this two-part breathing, combining abdomen and rib movement, three or four times. Then bring breathing back to normal and relax.

Finally: Place your hands on your collarbone, exhale fully, and inhale, feeling the abdomen expand, the rib cage open, and the collarbone rise. On exhalation, the collarbone rises slightly, rib cage contracts, and abdomen pulls back. (Once you've learned it, you can place your hands on your lap.)

When you put it all together, you're doing deep three-part breathing. Practice deep three-part breathing for three minutes a day. "People often see positive benefits right away," says Scheller. "You're bringing in much more oxygen. And when you breathe deeply, it helps release muscle tension. A heart patient often is unaware that he has tension in the body and constriction in the vessels. The best thing about the breathing is that it can be done anywhere. If you get hit with a stressful situation, and start the deep breathing, it may counteract any harmful effects of stress."

There is one precaution. If you start feeling dizzy or

light-headed, it's a signal that your brain can't handle so much oxygen. Stop and bring your breathing back to normal. It may take a few days to work up to 3 minutes. Aim to spend at least 20 minutes a day on yoga stretching and breathing.

Meditation

You may want to try meditation immediately after the three-part breathing. Find a quiet place. Sit on a chair or the floor, with your spine straight; a firm cushion under your buttocks should make you more comfortable on the floor.

There are many ways to meditate. You can focus on your breathing, simply concentrating on it. You can focus on a word or sound, repeating it silently on the out breath; some people use "Peace," "Relax," or "Love," or words from their faith, like "Hail Mary, full of grace" or "Shalom." For some, a relaxing image works best.

At times, your attention will wander. That's part of the process. Simply bring it back to your focus, and don't get discouraged. In time, you'll feel profound relaxation as you meditate.

It's best to meditate at the same time and place every day. Wait a few hours after eating. Aim to do it every day, even if you can only last a minute. If you persist, you'll find you can sit longer. In time, work up to at least one 20-minute sitting each day.

Group Support

Work on improving communications with your family and friends, or if you're feeling isolated, on finding ways to get involved with other people.

Dr. Ornish believes that opening up to others and communicating better helps heart patients get well. "Can you do it on your own? Yes. Is it easier if you have a group? Yes. But it doesn't have to be a group of heart patients," he says. "It can be any kind of group. The idea is to be in a group that feels safe enough for you to show who you really are under the masks and defenses, and rather than feeling rejected, feel supported. That in itself is healing."

CHAPTER 10

A New Weapon against Alcoholism

The strength of family and friends is a powerful tool for getting people into the treatment they need.

Jack Williams, 58, a successful insurance executive with an infectious laugh and a reputation for giving people the shirt off his back, stood over the hamburgers at the family's country home near San Antonio, Texas. Williams was in charge of the barbecue at the college graduation celebration he and his wife, Claire, were giving their son, Andy. He swatted flies, flipped hamburgers, and glanced at his watch. "It's five o'clock somewhere in the world," he said. "It must be time for a drink. Beer anyone?"

Actually, Jack had begun the morning with several Bloody Marys. His early afternoon "Cokes" were surreptitiously spiked with vodka from a stash in the trunk of his car. Claire, an attractive, youthful 55-year-old, eyed him warily. His speech was slurred. She felt her stomach tighten.

Claire couldn't help eavesdropping on Jack and their 21-

year-old son, Andy. Andy wanted to borrow $25 until he got his paycheck the following day. "No!" Jack shouted. "Not only no, but hell no!" Embarrassed, Andy stomped off with a group of his friends. By dinnertime, Jack weaved as he walked from the barbecue to the picnic table with a platter of burgers. Slurring his words, he yelled, "Cum'n get emmm!"

His brother-in-law Billy said to him quietly, "Hey Jack, don't you think you've had enough to drink?"

"Kiss my butt," Jack yelled belligerently. "Don't you tell me who's had too much."

"Grandad, these hamburgers are all bloody in the middle," 12-year-old Heather said, disappointed.

"You don't like 'em? Jes' throw 'em away," Jack retorted with a sneer to the granddaughter he often called "the best girlfriend in my life."

Then, on his way to get more pickles and beer, Jack tripped over a garden hose. The family stared in embarrassment as he struggled to pick himself up off the lawn. Finally, he passed out in the hammock, an aluminum can propped by his side. "Well, honey," his daughter, Linda, drawled to Claire, "chalk this up as another unforgettable party for the happy Williams family."

The next morning Jack bounced downstairs, pecked Claire on the cheek, and merrily chirped, "One hell of a party last night, huh?" He'd repressed all traces of the misery he'd caused his family.

"Oh God, what am I going to do?" Claire whispered to herself. The action Claire took saved her family—and probably her husband's life. She barely heard the announcement on the morning television show, but the dreaded word "alcoholism" caught her attention and she ran into the family room to listen.

"Don't wait till he kills himself or someone else on the freeway," intoned the TV announcer. The segment was devoted to "intervention," a process that empowers loved ones to confront alcohol abusers and urge them into treatment. After careful rehearsal and planning sessions with alcoholism counselors, family members surprise alcoholic loved ones when they are sober and nonjudgmentally confront them about their drinking. The family provides treatment alternatives and a list of iron-clad consequences if the drinking doesn't stop.

Tears welled in Claire's eyes. She had nagged, yelled, pleaded, and threatened for 20 years, but nothing had stopped Jack's alcoholism. His drinking had steadily grown worse. Claire still had nightmares from the harrowing drive home from Sue and Bobby's recent anniversary party. Andy's ruined graduation bash was the last straw.

Hands trembling, Claire called the San Antonio Council on Alcoholism. She spoke with counselors Joan Ellis and Rod Radle, and took the first step toward healing her family.

Session 1: The Problem

They sat on well-worn sofas in the counselors' group room: Claire; son Andy, a tall, slightly awkward young man; daughter Linda, 35, a carbon copy of her mother; and Linda's 12-year-old daughter, Heather. The room had a comfortable living room feel, complete with beige carpeting, potted plants in baskets, and a wicker coffee table covered with magazines. A cozy setting, but the topic they were about to tackle was not so cozy.

Counselor Joan Ellis, a woman with a take-charge manner, introduced herself and her partner, Rod, a rangy six-footer who lounged comfortably back in his chair. "We are licensed professional counselors, specialists in the field of alcohol abuse. We'd like to know what brings you here."

Claire and Linda sighed. Andy and Heather laughed nervously. Claire explained they wanted to confront Jack about his alcoholism. "Tell us what's been going on in your family," Ellis and Radle said. A familiar litany unfolded. "Thirty years ago," Claire said, "I sat on my Daddy's bed, him into his second bottle of bourbon, and vowed I'd never marry an alcoholic. But I did. How could I have done that?

"Jack was drunk when I met him," Claire continued. "It was at a party." She recounted the pattern. Daily drinking in the evenings and beginning early on weekends. The distance between them had grown, the communication lessened. Family fighting and bickering became constant.

To Contact
an Alcoholism Counselor

The best news for families struggling with alcoholism is that plenty of help is available. If you need help from a counselor, look for one who is specifically trained in alcoholism intervention. Local alcoholism agencies, your family physician, friends and acquaintances, or the psychology, counseling, or social work departments at local universities may be able to provide referrals. You can also contact the following organizations to find counselors near you.

National Association of Children of Alcoholics
(NACOA)
31706 Coast Highway
South Laguna, CA 92677
(714) 499-3889

Al-Anon Family Group Headquarters
P. O. Box 182
Madison Square Station
New York, NY 10159

Alcoholics Anonymous (AA)
468 Park Avenue
New York, NY 10016
(212) 686-1100

Women for Sobriety
Box 618
Quakertown, PA 18951
(215) 636-8026

Special occasions had become an excuse for drinking and an embarrassing time for the family. Then there was the time Jack had a car accident, but wasn't picked up for driving while intoxicated. And the time he got into a fight with a local grocery store manager.

"How could I have married an alcoholic?" Claire asked again rhetorically. The answer emerged in the family tree Ellis drew on a newsprint pad. Like most families of alcoholics, Claire's had a long history of alcoholism. Children, grandchildren, nieces, and nephews often unconsciously repeat the pattern either by becoming alcoholics or marrying them, or both.

Ellis and Radle gave the family members "homework" for the following week's session. Each person was to write a list of incidents detailing Jack's drinking behavior.

Session 2: The Incidents

"How's everybody been feeling this week?" Ellis asked.

Claire sighed, "I've been feeling like I'm lining up my bullets, but not to kill, to heal. I don't like bullets."

"You feel like a persecutor?"

"Yes."

"And our telling you that you're doing the right thing to save your husband—doesn't that help?"

"Yes, yes it does."

"Claire, there's a part of you that knows it's very important to tell Jack these things."

"Yes, but I feel like I'm blowing up Heather's world, saying all these things in front of her. And Andy is already so angry. It's like I'm giving him more ammunition to be angry and defeating my purpose."

Turning to Heather, Ellis asked, "Is your grandmother blowing up your world?"

"Kinda, but I don't blame her." Heather fidgeted and leaned closer to her mother.

"It's like there has been this secret all these years," Ellis explained, "and now your grandmother is saying we have to talk about Jack's disease. It's the only thing she can do to save his life, but she's scared about upsetting you."

"Let's review what we're doing," said Ellis. "You're

confronting your family's denial and creating a crisis for Jack. You're the ones who have been in crisis all these years. And in order for him to change, he must face a crisis. This family could wait another five or ten years and let him create his own crisis. Or wait for him to run off the freeway or run over a ten-year-old. That was the old way, waiting for the alcoholic to hit rock bottom, have a car accident, and kill someone. Intervention is another way. Moving the bottom up, creating a crisis for the alcoholic by giving evidence and fact. You don't have to wait till he kills someone."

Radle added, "You are saying to your husband, father, and grandfather, we love you and want to help you."

"My friend, Ann, asked me last night," Claire said, " 'Are you waiting until Jack kills someone?' "

"What was your answer?" asked Ellis.

"I told her I'm not waiting any longer."

Heather fidgeted and breathed deeply.

"Heather, can you tell us how you're feeling about all this?" asked Radle.

"It's like a lump in my throat that won't go away," she answered plaintively. "Is he really this bad off?"

"Yes, he is," answered Radle. "Your grandfather is sick. He has a disease. He's out of control and can't help himself. Unlike other people who can drink and not have a problem, something about his makeup causes him to be addicted to alcohol."

"I want to help him," said Heather, groping for her mother's hand.

Claire reached into her purse for the two sheets of rumpled paper that was her homework. She cleared her throat. "Jack, I've loved you from the first minute I laid eyes on you. You've given me everything I ever wanted—our precious children, our home. I love you very much and want you to be well. I'm convinced now that you have a disease and I want to help you. Remember last summer at Canyon Lake? We'd taken the kids waterskiing and you were drunk by noon. I was so scared when you drove the boat. I was afraid you might hit a skier. And on the drive home, the car was weaving off the road. When I asked you to let me drive, you yelled at me that I was a pushy bitch. Jack, I know you wouldn't have acted like that if you hadn't been drinking," Claire sighed.

"Good example," Ellis said. She moved to the newsprint and wrote "Canyon Lake, boat and car driving erratic." "What we'll do now is list everyone's incidents and choose the ones with the most impact. This is a good one." she said.

"Claire, let's back up and be more specific," Radle said. "Exactly when was this incident—June, July?—and how did you know he was drunk? Be specific. We can't leave any room for Jack to deny this." Claire pursed her lips, turned to the family. They pinpointed the date. They concluded they knew he was drunk because his speech was slurred, he swayed when he walked, and he acted belligerent.

"Okay Claire, any more incidents?"

Laughing nervously, Claire said, "I didn't realize it would be so hard to remember. There was the time in December of 1987 when . . ."

Claire finished her list. Linda opened her notebook and began to read her litany of incidents. Then Andy. Finally Heather. Ellis compiled the list of ten incidents. Each incident included the same points—a clear statement of how the family knew Jack was drunk, the date, and statements of love and concern. The mood changed from apprehension to seriousness. The family was working together. The mood grew lighter as it became safer to talk about Jack's addiction.

Session 3: Treatment Alternatives

"I'm just not willing to divorce Jack," Claire said during the family's discussion of treatments and consequences. "We've decided if he won't go to AA, then there's outpatient help, and that the last resort is hospitalization."

"I can't go through with a court commitment order," Andy said.

"That's okay, we can," Claire and Linda agreed.

"We're all worried about what happens after the intervention," Linda said, expressing the family's fears about following through with the consequences they'd discussed.

"It's important to be able to follow through with your consequences," Radle said. "It will be worse than before if you can't. More harm than good. But remember, you carry a lot of power with the love and facts you will be presenting to him. You're building such a tight case he won't be able to argue with you."

Ellis added. "The bottom line is that after you go through with this intervention, he may not change, at least not right away. But statistics show that 90 percent of alcoholics confronted this way begin treatment of some sort.

"What's happening in your family is that you are all taking control for the first time. You are talking to Jack about his drinking and saying, if you drink, number one we're going to talk about it and number two we're prepared to take action."

"Did you find out about hospitalization?" Radle asked.

"Yes," Claire replied. "I called the insurance people and they said alcoholism is a disease like any other and both hospitalization and counseling are covered."

"What you have to do is make Jack want to stop drinking," Radle said. "Right now, the way it is in your family, he can keep on drinking. He can say, 'I don't want to stop.' He's in control. So instead of bending over backward to make things nice, you're bending over backward to make it hard for him to drink. It's the only way you're going to help."

Rehearsal

"Let's talk about where to have the session and how you're going to get him there," Ellis and Radle said, insisting the confrontation occur at a time when Jack was sober. The family decided they couldn't get Jack to come to the counselors' office. He knew they were coming to counseling every Wednesday evening, but his response was always, "You guys have a problem, not me."

"We'll tell him his insurance agent has to see him on Saturday morning," Linda suggested.

"No, let's tell him Heather wants him to take her to North Star Mall Saturday morning," Andy said.

"We can't lie to him," explained Radle. "It's very important to be straightforward and not give him any excuse to walk out on us."

The family settled on doing the intervention at home. Jack liked big Saturday morning breakfasts before disappearing into his woodworking shop, so they agreed to be up and ready by eight o'clock. When he came downstairs, Linda was selected to say, "Dad, we have invited some friends over and we'd all like just an hour of your time. Please join us in the living room." Ellis and Radle promised to be there.

"If he's in his own home, he'll be less likely to bolt," Radle said.

"Oh God, what if he gets mad?" cried Linda.

"Quietly repeat that you just want an hour of his time. Put your hand gently on his arm, look him directly in the eye. Be kind and firm," Radle said.

"He's going to be a pussycat," Claire decided. "I just know it. I know because I've felt calmer and calmer. I don't feel so afraid anymore."

"That's because you finally understand his illness," Ellis said.

"Who's going to go first," asked Radle, "and where is everyone going to sit?"

"We've decided Linda should lead off," said Claire. "We think Jack will respond best to her, Daddy's little girl and all. Then Andy, then me, and we'll end up with Heather, which should really finish him off."

Andy leaned over to read what Linda had written for her opening and burst out laughing. "I can't help it," he said, trying to control himself. "It sounds just like a Hallmark card."

Linda grinned at him. "Yeah, some of us have all the talent." Claire and Heather joined Andy's chuckling. The laughter relieved their tension.

The family discussed seating: Dad in his easy chair; Linda to his right; Claire to the left; and Andy and Heather on either side. Ellis and Radle would sit behind Claire toward the back. They explained that their role during intervention was to be supportive and ready to aid, but not to become actively involved unless necessary.

"But what if he says that's not the way it happened?" asked Heather.

"Linda will remind him that you are asking for an hour of his time to listen to you," answered Ellis. "And besides, this rarely happens. However, remember you are dealing with a toxic person and the manner in which you present this renders him pretty defenseless. If by chance he leaves, then the family will simply put all of this in writing."

The family positioned themselves as they would for Saturday morning. Radle, his face serious, "played" Jack. Linda began, "Dad, I love you very much. You've always been there for me." Tears streamed down her face. "I can't get through this without crying."

"Tears are fine," Ellis explained. "They are an expression of caring. If you can't continue, Andy will do his part and we'll come back to you. You can look to us for support."

"I can do it," she said, smiling weakly. "Let me start over."

"Before you start, be sure to look me in the eye," said Radle. "Eye contact is all important. And I know this is hard, but try not to sound like you're reading. Say it from the heart."

The rehearsal continued. On the final run-through, there were no hitches, few tears. The Williamses were ready.

Intervention

Parking the car a few doors down from the Williamses' house, Ellis and Radle arrived promptly at 8:00 A.M. "I always get the feeling it's opening night," commented Ellis about the palpable preintervention tension in the air. "We thought we'd lost him," a worried Claire whispered as she greeted the counselors. "He was so bad last night. Belligerent. Threatening to take off driving. This morning he's fine and upstairs dressing."

Linda bounced to the front door, shaking her hands in nervousness. "I'll be okay if we can just get started," she said.

The family took their positions. Linda stood tensely,

Alcoholism:
Our Number One Drug
Problem

Forget about crack, cocaine, speed, and heroin. Alcohol is the most widely abused drug in North America and alcoholism is the number one drug problem. Upward of 20 million people in the United States drink to excess (14 or more drinks a week). According to the National Council on Alcoholism, 12 million of these people have one or more symptoms of alcoholism.

Alcoholism is the third largest killer in North America and would probably be number one if blood alcohol levels were determined for all victims of suicide, homicide, accidents, and car wrecks.

Although alcoholism varies from person to person, the disease begins with social drinking. Then come episodes of binges or weekend drunks. The alcoholic develops a tolerance and requires more drinks to stay high. Personality changes occur. The shy, dependent person may become abusively aggressive when drunk. The pleasant, easygoing friend may become despondent and depressed with alcohol. Relationships with the alcoholic deteriorate. Denial is a theme throughout the progression of the disease. "You have a problem, not me" is a consistent alcoholic reply. Then deception begins—sneaking drinks, hiding stashes of liquor, becoming angry if drinking time is cut short.

In 1956, the American Medical Association named alcoholism a disease, but its cause is still a mystery. We know that while one person develops a tolerance for methyl alcohol, another doesn't. According to Vernon Johnson, founder of the Johnson Institute in Minneapolis, a training and treatment center for chemical dependency, because drinking is so prevalent and socially acceptable in this country, "anyone in America who can, will become an alcoholic."

Alcoholics gradually lose control over their drinking. Once addicted, no amount of reason or logic can stop it. Alcoholic self-destructive behavior is a mystery to family and friends. If they are suffering all these problems, why do they keep drinking? It's not that alcoholics want to drink, it's that they can't stop. They're addicted.

Alcoholism affects all walks of life, all social strata. A successful businessman like Jack is a more typical alcoholic than the stereotypic skid-row bum. Only about 3 percent of alcoholics fit the lying-in-the-gutter image. Because the disease is progressive, often taking years to develop, most alcoholics are able to maintain their jobs, though their family life may have disintegrated much earlier. Due to the disease's inherent denial mechanism, even family and friends deny the problem—and thus delay help—until it's often too late.

chewing one side of her mouth. Claire watched the stairway, her eyes unblinking. Andy tried deep breathing and Heather sat swinging her feet. Finally, Jack, whistling, bounded down the stairs, "Hey, where is everybody?"

Trying not to appear too curious, Ellis and Radle glanced at Jack, the man this family had been so afraid to confront. Tall, trim, smelling of shaving lotion, the epitome of the successful businessman. There was no physical hint of his illness, except some telltale puffiness under his eyes.

Linda, touching her hand to her chest to still her racing heart, began, "Dad?" Surprised, cautious but polite, Jack nodded at Ellis and Radle, but quickly turned to the family. "What's going on here?"

"Dad, please sit down. Just promise you'll give us an hour of your time," the words tumbled from Linda. Jack remained silent while Linda talked. Tears streamed down her face, but her voice was steady until she finished her rehearsed part. Jack listened without expression.

Then quickly, Andy began. "Dad, I love you very much and I want to help you." He choked, then continued. "At my graduation party in August, we had all gathered to celebrate. You were cooking for us all, but I knew you'd been drinking by the way you were slurring your words. I know you wouldn't have yelled at me in front of my friends if you hadn't been drinking. Dad, if you'll stop drinking, we can have our family back again. I can have my Dad back."

The tension in the room was electric but controlled. The rehearsal had paid off. Jack, perhaps sensing the power of these undeniable facts so lovingly offered, appeared mesmerized, in shock. As in a well-rehearsed play, there were no pauses, no hesitations. But unlike a play, the tears were real.

Heather spoke, first in her little-girl voice, then warming up and becoming stronger. "Grandad, you mean my life to me. I wish you would stop drinking. I remember last year at my birthday party, I waited and waited, but you didn't come until after my party was over. I could smell the liquor on your breath and you stumbled around, talking loud. I felt so bad. Grandad, I think you have a drinking problem."

Jack took off his glasses, fidgeted, then rose to leave. "This is enough," he said quietly.

"Dad, please, you promised us an hour," Linda said. She looked him in the eye, and gently seated him. "Before we go on, is there anything you'd like to say to us?"

Jack pursed his lips. He began to shake his head. His face wore a mask of surprise and anguish. "Well, happy Saturday morning to you all, too." The silence from the family was deafening. Jack finally said, "I know everything you say is true. I had no idea I'd hurt you all so much."

"Dad, we're almost through. First we want to tell you about help that is available. We want you to know it's your choice. First, there's Alcoholics Anonymous along with some form of individual counseling. Second would be outpatient treatment. Third, there are some very good hospital programs in San Antonio for this problem."

Claire straightened her shoulders, breathed in, and delivered the clincher. "Jack, with all the love we feel for you, we must tell you that if you don't stop drinking, we are prepared to ask you to leave this house." Her voice was calm and strong. "And Jack, we are prepared to have you hospitalized."

Jack slumped forward and released a loud sob. "Oh God, help me. What have I done to you? Please help me." He put a hand on his forehead and said repeatedly, "I had no idea . . . I never would have . . ." Finally Jack composed himself, carefully removed his handkerchief from his pocket, and slowly, deliberately wiped his eyes. "This is very sudden. Do I have to decide today? And these people," he said, nodding toward Ellis and Radle, "they'll think I'm a falling-down drunk."

Claire, in a firm, kind voice, replied, "Jack, these counselors helped us prepare for today. They've helped us understand alcoholism and how it is a disease over which you have no control. Don't feel embarrassed. They are helping us save your life." Claire swallowed hard and continued. "We must have your commitment today, Jack, to quit drinking. We understand you need time to think about the form of treatment. But we expect an answer by tomorrow or Monday or we are prepared to follow through with our consequences."

Ellis waited until Jack's sobs subsided and introduced herself and Radle and their specialty in alcohol abuse. "It was very difficult for your family to prepare for today, and I know you see it was done with a lot of love," said Ellis. She explained that she and Radle would help with follow-up treatment for the family and for him if he wanted. After leaving their phone number and the local number for Alcoholics Anonymous, they finally exited amid hugs from the family.

On leaving, the counselors heard Jack say, "I don't want to go to a hospital. I don't want everybody to know." His voice sounded soft, hesitating. "Will you call AA for me?"

Outside, Ellis and Radle breathed a collective sigh of relief and said in unison, "Whew!" The Williamses had finally broken the alcoholic code of silence and taken control of the disease.

Is Your Child
at Risk for Alcoholism?

The statistics are frightening: 65 percent of high-school seniors say they drink and 39 percent drink five or more drinks in a row once or twice every weekend. Harmless kid stuff? Probably not, according to William C. Van Ost, M.D., and Elaine Van Ost, coauthors of *Warning Signs: A Parent's Guide to In-Time Intervention in Drug and Alcohol Abuse*.

"Adolescence is a tough time," they write. "Plagued by everything from being turned down for dates to uncertainty about careers, teenagers agonize over momentary setbacks and lifetime decisions." The coauthors contend teenagers are especially vulnerable to drinking due to peer pressure, thrill seeking, and pro-drug/alcohol messages in the media.

Often, the Van Osts say, parents are unaware their child has an alcohol problem until the situation escalates into a crisis. They suggest seeking help if you notice any of the following warning signs.

- Noticeably lower levels in liquor bottles kept at home.
- The smell of alcohol in cups, glasses, or open soda cans.
- Bottles in unlikely places around the house.
- Empty bottles of extracts such as vanilla that have high alcohol levels.
- Changes in the child's friends.
- Personality changes.
- Deteriorating grades or absences from school.
- Missing money or personal belongings.

In addition to these warning signs, the authors suggest evaluating your child's risk for becoming alcoholic through the use of "genograms," outlines of

> family trees that trace alcohol abuse among family members. Since a family history of alcoholism is a strong risk factor for the disease, recognizing the special risk relatives of alcoholics face is a valuable tool in prevention.

Follow-Up

The Williamses attended a follow-up session on Monday. Although Jack was invited, he chose not to attend. Each member evaluated the intervention, ventilated feelings, and discussed what to do if Jack were to resume drinking.

"Let's talk about what if," said Radle, reminding the family of their commitment to follow through on their consequences. "Jack has been told, if you drink again, this will happen." Radle reassured the family that the counselors would be available for continued sessions and assistance.

"You're not just hanging us out to dry," laughed Claire.

"No," answered Ellis. "This is the beginning of a process. The beginning of your family getting well. Jack built up a tolerance for alcohol, but the family built up a tolerance for his alcoholic behavior. You will now be able to say, 'Jack, I see you are drinking. Our arrangement is that if you drink, you cannot stay in this house. I love you and I'm disappointed and would prefer that you let me help you get help.' "

"We've decided to go to Al-Anon," said Claire, referring to the organization modeled after AA for the families of alcoholics.

"We couldn't recommend it more," smiled Ellis.

"And the real key is follow-through," Radle said. "You must be willing to remind Jack of the treatment alternatives, but then be willing to follow through with your consequences." Radle continued discussing what-ifs and one by one the family rehearsed their agreed-on alternatives.

"I feel a little let down and depressed after all this," admitted Linda. "The thrill is gone and it's not just 'poof!'

all better. The important thing is that now I know what to say and what to do."

"I said things to my father I never believed I'd ever be able to say," mused Andy. "I was always afraid he'd put me down or say I didn't know what I was talking about. But I see that if we can talk to our father, it will help us talk to one another and to our friends."

"Yes," concluded Radle, "you are all on the way to health. Removing alcohol has given this family a chance."

CHAPTER 11

Walk Your Way to Wellness

Current research is showing that increased fitness levels extend lives.

To most of us, a prescription is something we get from the doctor and take to the pharmacist. It's medicine we get when we're ill. We take it for a while and stop when we're better.

Well, here's a prescription for nearly everyone—sick or well. To get the maximum effect, you should continue to take it for the rest of your life. It's a remedy backed by the most knowledgeable and respected physicians in the world . . .

Rx: Start a regular walking program and stay with it.

Fill this prescription right away, and you may begin to notice some very impressive benefits.

The latest studies have made it official: Even a low to moderately intense level of physical activity—such as walking—can reduce your odds of falling victim to a whole host of life-threatening diseases. Not only that, but the years you add can be healthy, productive, and enjoyable, thanks to an increased level of fitness.

Some of the strongest evidence for the health-enhancing effect of moderate exercise, including walking, comes from a long-term study recently published in the *Journal of the American Medical Association*. Data for the study were gathered over 11 years at the Institute for Aerobics Research, in Dallas. The researchers used a standard treadmill test to determine the physical fitness of 13,344 people. Then each person was assigned to one of five fitness levels based on age, sex, and treadmill-endurance time. All the study participants underwent a full medical examination. At the time of enrollment in the study, none of them had ever had a heart attack, stroke, chronic high blood pressure, or diabetes.

Over the follow-up period (8 to 19 years per person, depending on the time of enrollment), 283 people in the group died. When the primary cause of death and any contributing causes were matched with the fitness ranking, there were some real surprises. The overall rate of death for the least fit men was nearly 3½ times higher than that of the most fit men. For the least fit women, the death rate was over 4½ times higher than that for the most fit women.

Even more eye-opening in women, the risk of death for the next-to-lowest fitness group was only about 50 percent of the risk of dying among the lowest fitness group. In men, the next-to-lowest ranking had about 40 percent of the death rate of the lowest. That's a dramatic reduction in risk for a relatively low to moderate level of fitness.

The suggestion of this and other research? Even a very modest walking program may provide impressive health benefits if you've been inactive in the past. If you're already somewhat active, a regular walking program can help increase your fitness level.

Rx:

- The walking prescription for general good health, as outlined by the researchers in this study, is to take a brisk walk of 30 to 60 minutes per day. That's an ideal schedule designed to maintain a fairly high standard of physical fitness.
- The recommended minimum amount of walking, based on numerous other studies, seems to be 20 minutes,

done briskly, at least three times per week. This will maintain a moderate level of fitness. But as we said, any exercise is better than none at all.

● Walking for more than 60 minutes per day doesn't seem to add much to overall risk reduction. So fanaticism carries no additional health benefits.

You Can Lower
Your Heart Disease Risk

If you don't get any exercise, your chances of having a heart attack are more than tripled, according to studies from the University of North Carolina at Chapel Hill. The studies were similar to those mentioned above: 3,106 healthy men and 2,802 healthy women were assigned fitness ratings based on treadmill results. The follow-up revealed a higher death rate from cardiovascular disease for people in the lowest level of fitness. No real surprise there. But the results held up even after adjusting for other risks such as age, smoking, cholesterol level, and high blood pressure.

This means the studies confirm earlier research showing that a lack of fitness is itself a major independent risk factor for heart disease. To put that risk in perspective, the Chapel Hill researchers point out that an inactive person's risk of heart disease is the same as that of someone who smokes a pack of cigarettes a day.

The good news is that there are several ways that walking helps your heart. The most direct is by exercising the heart itself, which is a muscle. Other ways involve helping to reduce excess weight, high blood pressure, bad cholesterol ratios, and diabetic symptoms. (More on these in a minute.)

Rx:

● The walking prescription for heart health is a minimum of 20 minutes of brisk walking at least three times per week. Better yet, walk every day. Once around the block is fine to start, but it'll only get you so far, fitness-wise as well as distance-wise.

- Let your physician advise you of a safe target pulse rate for your exercise.
- Even if you're subject to angina attacks—the chest pains associated with heart disease—you may be able to safely begin a walking program. But it must be done under a doctor's supervision, in a medically supervised setting, if possible, especially if you take medication. (The doctor may recommend monitoring pulse rate on the basis of a stress test if you have heart disease.) At the first sign of a problem, see your personal physician.
- If you have a history of angina, don't walk with hand weights and avoid walking in very cold weather, especially if it's windy. Also, don't carry anything weighing more than a few ounces on long fitness walks. Any added strain on the upper extremities can trigger chest pain. If you have chest pain when walking, *stop*—call your doctor immediately. Don't continue your walking program until you've discussed the pain with him. If you have been prescribed nitroglycerin, make sure you have it with you.

You Can Alter Your Cholesterol Profile

Today, virtually everyone has heard of the dangers of high blood cholesterol. Walking probably won't do much to lower your overall blood cholesterol level. But it may do something just as important: raise your high-density lipo-protein (HDL) cholesterol. High HDL levels are associated with a lower risk of heart disease.

Walking may even protect against heart disease despite stubbornly high cholesterol levels, at least in men. In the Institute for Aerobics Research study, men with high over-all cholesterol who scored in the top two fitness levels had less than half the risk of death of men with low overall cholesterol who scored in the lowest fitness level. In other words, even low cholesterol provides less heart disease protection if you're unfit.

Rx:

- The walking prescription for raising protective HDL levels is the same as that for lowering heart disease risks.

You Can Control
High Blood Pressure

There's good evidence that some people can control their mildly high blood pressure simply by maintaining a regular exercise program. That's a big plus because many blood pressure–lowering medications have negative side effects. Even those who still need medication may be able to lower their dosage if they exercise.

Regular walking is a good exercise for hypertension because unlike, say, a spirited game of one-on-one basketball, walking won't raise already high blood pressure to dangerous levels. Yet walking gives the cardiovascular system a workout, promoting greater efficiency and lowering blood pressure. Also, since weight gain often triggers high blood pressure, the gradual loss of weight through a regular walking program is an additional way to bring blood pressure down.

A good level of fitness may have other protective benefits for hypertensives, even in cases where it doesn't lower blood pressure. In the Institute for Aerobics Research study, both men and women in the top two fitness levels suffering from high blood pressure had a much lower rate of death than people in the bottom fitness level with low blood pressure. As with cholesterol, a good reading on the blood pressure scale may mean a lot less if you're out of shape.

Rx:

The walking prescription for high blood pressure is similar to the program recommended for heart disease protection, with the following precautions:

- If you're hypertensive, don't use hand weights to increase your walking workout. Exercising your leg muscles won't raise your blood pressure significantly during exercise. But additional exercise of the smaller muscles in your arms can raise your blood pressure, sometimes to dangerous levels.
- If you're taking any antihypertensive medication, talk with your doctor before beginning a walking program or other exercise. There are many different types of

blood pressure medication, so find out from your physician the particular side effects or warning signs to watch for in your case. And set up a regular schedule of visits to monitor your progress. Don't change the dosage of any of your medicines without your doctor's approval.

- Walking up even relatively steep grades should cause you no harm. But take it slowly at first and use common sense.

You Can Lose Weight

Obesity is one of the top health problems in this country. Even a little excess weight increases your risk of cardiovascular problems, high blood pressure, diabetes, and a host of other ills.

Dieting can help some people lose weight, but most dieters tend to get trapped in an endless lose/gain cycle. That's partly because they're only attacking one end of the problem. They try to control their calorie intake, but forget about their calorie outgo. Fact is, you can lose weight by increasing the number of calories you burn without changing your intake—that is, without dieting (although anyone trying to lose weight should start a sensible, low-calorie eating plan). If more overweight people thought of themselves not as overeaters but as underexercisers, there'd be a lot more thin people in the world.

Rx:

- The walking prescription for weight loss is more immediately concerned with the number of calories burned during exercise than in aerobic fitness, although ideally the two eventually go hand-in-hand. For that reason, it's less crucial to keep up the pace and more important to make sure that you meet a goal of, say, 3 to 5 miles on a daily basis. Even if you can only manage a half mile to start, walking every day gets you in the habit.
- To figure out how you're doing, here's a simple equation: If you walk at the leisurely pace of 3 miles per hour (1 mile every 20 minutes), you can burn up to 300 calories an hour. Do that every day, and you can lose 2 pounds per month with no change in diet. Combine that with a

300-calorie-per-day cut in food intake, and you can drop 4 pounds per month! Cutting food intake is a challenge, though: Exercise increases appetite.

- If you move at the brisker pace of 4 miles per hour, you'll burn about 400 to 500 calories per hour. If the terrain is hilly or you walk faster, you'll burn a bit more than that. These are estimates, of course. The actual number of calories you expend will vary slightly according to the distance you walk, the type of terrain (hilly or flat), fluctuations in your pace, and your weight.
- By comparison, jogging burns only about 20 percent more calories than brisk walking. But compare how you feel at the end of a 3-mile walk with how you feel when you jog that same distance. Jogging may take more out of you if you're overweight. With less chance of injury and fatigue, even out-of-shape people can exercise longer and more frequently by walking. That translates into a greater number of calories burned.
- If you're more than 20 pounds overweight and you've been inactive for a while, make a point to get good-quality walking shoes before you start exercising. Look for good arch support and plenty of toe room. Good shoes are important for all exercise walkers, but even more so for inactive people with a lot of weight to lose. People carrying a lot of excess weight are more prone to overuse injuries, such as plantar fasciitis (a common cause of heel pain), and general circulation problems in the legs and feet.
- If you're 50 or more pounds overweight, seek a doctor's advice before beginning any exercise program, even walking. If you get chest pains during exercise or have chronic foot or leg problems, consult your personal physician.

You Can Control Diabetes

Diabetes can be triggered by weight gain in adulthood. And diabetes can put you at greater risk of developing cardiovascular disease. These problems may be reduced with a regular walking plan.

Here's how: First, exercise and weight loss make the body more sensitive to levels of insulin naturally released through the bloodstream. This allows the body to better control the blood sugar level. Second, by burning energy at a steady rate, walking increases the muscles' demand for glucose, helping to clear excess sugar from the bloodstream. Both these effects can benefit insulin-dependent diabetics as well.

In someone taking insulin, a significantly more vigorous activity than walking could clear too much sugar from the bloodstream too quickly. That might lead to hypoglycemic attacks.

Rx:

The walking prescription for diabetes is more moderately paced than that for heart disease prevention. Diabetics get greater benefits from several low-intensity walks per day. Instead of one hour-long walk daily, try two or three 20- to 30-minute walks per day, preferably after meals. Take care to follow several important precautions:

- Before beginning any sort of workout, go to your doctor for a checkup. If your blood sugar control is good, you should still be checked for peripheral vascular disease (PVD) and nerve damage in your feet and legs. People over 30 or those who've been diabetic for more than 15 years may need to have an electrocardiogram/treadmill test to check for early heart disease.
- Also before beginning your walking program, get an ophthalmologic exam to determine if you have retinopathy. (Regular eye exams, of course, are important whether you exercise or not.) If present, this condition can get worse when pressure in the eye increases, which may happen during exertion. If you've got it, you may have to take extra precautions to preserve your sight.
- Proper walking shoes are a must! Don't buy them off the bargain rack. Go to a reputable store and have them fitted. Take along the socks you'll be wearing during exercise. Make sure the shoe is snug but not tight over the sock, with plenty of room for the toes to move around. A removable insole is good since some people with PVD or other foot problems need to use orthotics

(special molded shoe inserts). If in doubt, consult your podiatrist.

- A note about socks: Skip the all-cotton brands. They bunch up when wet and can cause blisters. Wool and synthetic blends are better. They provide warmth and wick moisture away from the feet.
- Inspect your feet frequently. You can rub a little petroleum jelly on chafing points of the feet to help prevent blisters. Tell your doctor about any blisters or skin ulcers that aren't healing properly.
- Dehydration can cause blood sugar problems, so it's wise to take a drink shortly before walking, especially on hot days. Milk or natural fruit juices may be better choices than water because they provide you with a little extra energy for the exercise period ahead.
- To counter episodes of hypoglycemia (low blood sugar) during a walk, people taking insulin should carry a few glucose tablets. They're better than a candy bar because they are more readily absorbable. Most pharmacies stock them, and they're available without a doctor's prescription.
- If you have insulin-dependent diabetes, you may be able to lower your insulin requirements after you've been on a walking program for a while. Don't try it on your own—stick to your physician's advice. You should carry an ID card or medic-alert bracelet in case of an emergency.

You Can Fight Osteoporosis

Research has shown that weight-bearing exercises like walking can have a protective effect against osteoporosis. In fact, some of the studies have compared exercise and calcium supplementation—and exercise won hands (and feet) down.

Most people forget that bone is living tissue. It might be more helpful if we thought of bone as something you can build up like muscle. And how do people build up muscle? Exercise! It's not quite that simple, of course. People with severe osteoporosis aren't going to build up their bones overnight. But for postmenopausal women who are at high risk, walking may be a good way to prevent (or at least slow down) bone demineralization. In one small year-long study from the USDA Human Nutrition Research Lab at Tufts University, nine postmenopausal women walked for 45 minutes a day, four days per week. (For eight months of the study, the women wore 8-pound waist weights while walking.) After a year, they showed a 3 percent increase in lower-spine bone density.

Three percent may not sound like much, but over the years it adds up. Inactive women of the same age range, who acted as experimental controls, had a 10 percent loss in bone density during the same period.

Rx:

- Though there's no proof that exercise decreases bone-fracture rates, the best walking prescription for osteoporosis prevention seems to be a 45-minute daily walk, four to six times per week. If you've already got osteoporosis, you can build up to that exercise level. Start out with 10-minute walks, three or four times per week. If that goes well, add 5 minutes per week until you reach 45 minutes per walk.
- If you have moderate to severe osteoporosis, or have recently broken a bone, you should check with your physician before beginning a walking program.
- You don't have to walk quickly. In fact, doing so could put you at greater risk for a fall . . . and a fracture. A moderate or even slow pace can strengthen bones safely.
- Be careful where you walk, to avoid falling. Hills, choppy pavement, gravel, and any other uneven surface can trip you up. Slippery surfaces and dark areas are also hazardous. Curtail solitary outdoor winter strolls and night walking. (Two good places to go for a walk: an indoor track and a mall.) Take along whatever support you need to keep your balance, such as a cane or a walker. Or try the buddy system. Leaning on a friend is fine (as long as the friend doesn't mind).
- Good walking shoes with plenty of cushion in the heel are important to minimize jarring and stress. The shoes should be comfortable, and you should feel like you can easily keep your balance in them.

You Can Feel Better and More in Control

One of the most overlooked benefits of exercise is the sense of well-being and control it can give you. And it's no illusion. If you're in good physical shape, you'll feel better, be more optimistic, and have higher self-esteem.

Walking is one of the best types of exercise from a psychological standpoint. It's not really competitive, so you can go at your own pace and feel good about it. Yet you can get a sense of accomplishment by going that extra mile, or finishing the usual course a minute quicker than last time. Walking gets you out into the world, whether you go outside or walk in a covered mall. You can walk alone when you want to spend time with your own thoughts. Or you can socialize by going out with one person or a whole group of people.

Would you believe walking may even act as a tranquilizer? In some studies done at California State University at Long Beach, preexam anxiety was significantly reduced in those students who took a brisk 10-minute walk. The researchers theorized that exercise can alter stress-related chemicals in the brain. Then, too, the physical activity of walking releases muscle tension. Don't discount the effect of pleasant surroundings along the walking path, either.

It's easy to listen to all the evidence and decide that walking is for you. It's not as easy to get out and actually start doing it. You may have to force yourself a little at first. But a walking program is a relatively simple prescription to follow, once you get used to it.

So what are you waiting for? You've got everything to gain and nothing to lose! Talk with your doctor if you have any doubts, and start taking your walking prescription today. If you stick with it, you may not need another prescription for a long, long time.

CHAPTER 12

Manage Diabetes Naturally

Tips from the American Diabetes Association help moti-vate the weight loss and exercise programs proven to extend diabetics' lives.

Three years ago, when she discovered she had diabetes, Margaret Moore was more scared than she'd ever been. "My blood sugar was so high [it was close to 700; normal is about 100] my doctor put me in the hospital right away. He said he wondered why I wasn't in a coma."

But today the 76-year-old Wichita schoolteacher sounds as chipper as she feels. "I have more energy, and I'm more clearheaded than I've been in years," she says. She's pared her weight down to normal and upgraded her diet to a careful selection of whole grains, fruits and vegetables, lean meats, low-fat dairy products, and beans. She manages to squeeze walks into her busy week. She's had none of the potentially fatal complications of diabetes. In fact, she says, "I feel like I could live to be 100."

Margaret Moore is an A-plus example of what's possible for people with Type II diabetes who are able and willing to assume responsibility for their own well-being. (Diabetes is the inability of the body to properly use and store blood sugar, or glucose. The food we eat is converted into glucose for use by the body. And Type II, the most common form of diabetes, is known as non-insulin-dependent diabetes mellitus. That's a bit of a misnomer, since about 25 percent of Type II's do require insulin injections to control their blood sugar, and 25 percent take oral drugs to increase insulin production and improve sugar metabolism.)

"People with Type II diabetes really have the opportunity to help control their own destiny," says Sherman Holvey, M.D., president of the American Diabetes Association (ADA). "The doctor may call the shots, but it's the patient who carries the ball. Weight management and exercise will pay off in better health and a longer life."

Using the Power of Pounds Off

Experts agree: Losing weight is by far the most effective way to treat Type II diabetes. It's the only thing many diabetics need to do to control their insulin and blood sugar.

Many Type II diabetics are 30 to 60 pounds overweight. For some, there's no question that losing just 10 pounds can make a big difference, says Robert Henry, M.D., a diabetes weight-loss specialist. After weight loss, all three major problems of Type II diabetes improve: Superhigh insulin levels drop; the liver, which has been secreting two to three times more sugar than normal into the blood, begins to produce less; and peripheral muscle tissues, previously resistant to the effect of insulin to enhance sugar uptake, take up sugar better.

"The most dramatic response to even a small weight loss is in diabetics whose insulin secretion is highest in the morning," Dr. Henry says. And people who've had diabetes five years or less respond best to weight loss. After that, it may become harder to control the disease by diet alone. Drugs may become necessary.

Some Type II diabetics become so insulin resistant they need to take additional insulin, or oral drugs that stimulate insulin production. These drugs can start a vicious circle that's hard to break. Studies show that insulin-treated diabetics tend to gain weight more often than diabetics who do not take insulin. That's because the additional insulin helps the body to metabolize, rather than excrete, sugar. Excess sugar is stored as body fat. And too much body fat makes diabetes worse.

If you must take medication but can still lose a few pounds, you may be able to cut back on your dosage gradually, with medical supervision.

Even when all these health-enhancing benefits of weight loss are crystal clear, and you're dead set on paring the pudge, you may still find it tough going. Here are some tactics you may not have heard about that could make the job a lot easier.

Make it so real you can see it. Many diabetics have failed to lose weight in the past and can't help but believe they're doomed to future failures. To break that way of thinking, diabetics need concrete advice on how to succeed, says Sheila Flood, R.N., a University of Rochester nutrition and behavior-modification educator who specializes in diabetes.

"We figure out exactly what each diabetic needs to do to lose weight, based on their weight and level of activity," she says. "I don't just say, 'You've got to cut calories.' I say, 'We can cut this 6-ounce T-bone steak down to 3 ounces and save 300 calories. Are you willing to do that?' I show them that riding a stationary bicycle for 10 minutes burns 60 calories, or that walking 1 mile burns 60 or 70 calories. We chisel off about 3,500 calories a week (1 pound) through diet and exercise. Diabetics learn that cutting a few calories here and burning a few calories there makes a tremendous difference. It's what puts them in control."

Mark your success by more than pounds. For many dieting diabetics, the carrot at the end of the stick isn't their ideal weight. It's whatever weight allows them to control their blood sugar well enough to completely eliminate or cut back drastically on their drug dosage or never have to take drugs in the first place. Monitoring the dramatic drops in blood sugar and cholesterol that accompany weight loss—rather than just watching the bathroom scale—helps people see that this worthy goal is attainable.

Beware of "diabetic" foods. Foods labeled "dietetic" or "diabetic" can be deceptive. It's true that they contain no sugar: They contain sorbitol, a lower-calorie sugar-alcohol. But some of these products are higher in fat and calories than their nondiabetic counterparts. Dietary fat, by the way, not only contributes to heart disease—it's also more easily converted into body fat than either carbohydrates or protein.

When it comes to sweets, know thyself. Some diabetics confess having a strong urge for sweets, an urge only made worse by total denial. Nutritionists offer this solution: If you know it's going to lead to bingeing, don't try to deprive yourself of sweets totally. Instead, incorporate controlled portions of sweets into your diet on a daily basis. Other diabetics, though, know they do better if they cut out all sweets except fruits. Why? Because they "can't eat just one." It's actually easier for them to go cold turkey than to fight temptation.

Plan a snack for your hungriest time. Four o'clock in the afternoon seems to be the bewitching hour for many would-be diabetic dieters. Their resistance to overeating drops to its lowest just about the time their insulin level is peaking. (Insulin is a well-known appetite stimulant; high insulin levels are thought to be one reason so many Type II diabetics struggle with weight loss.) The afternoon peak usually happens with naturally produced insulin (depending on when and what you've eaten so far during the day). And it happens like clockwork in people who take a morning injection of long-acting insulin and no other insulin during the day.

Instead of trying to stick it out and failing, plan a snack for this or any other particularly tempting time, says registered dietitian Christine Beebe, who specializes in diabetes management. Take the calories from somewhere else in your day. The trick is planning: It protects you from impulsively eating something you'd rather not.

Try a medically supervised low-calorie diet. If you're 10 to 30 pounds overweight, your best slimming scheme is simple: Reduce the number of calories in your normal diet. If you're more than 30 pounds overweight and have failed to lose weight because you can't stick to a 1,200- to 1,500-calorie diet, you may be more successful on a medically supervised low-calorie liquid diet, which quells most appetites.

"We use this to initiate weight loss," Dr. Henry says. "We might keep someone on it for a month, then gradually bring in foods that allow them to continue to lose weight, or maintain their weight loss." Diabetics need to be careful, though, or the pounds will creep back on.

Avoid weight-loss aids. Over-the-counter appetite suppressants that contain phenylpropanolamine (PPA) only compound a diabetic's problems. They can contribute to high blood pressure and kidney and eye problems. Taking thyroid drugs to lose weight can be trouble, too. While these drugs do take the weight off, a large amount of that lost weight is muscle, not fat. That can weaken the heart.

Learn to check your blood sugar. Type I (insulin-dependent) diabetics learn how to check their blood sugar; their lives depend on it! Many Type IIs, though, never learn. That's a mistake because monitoring blood sugar provides valuable information that can be used to adjust food or drug intake for all diabetics. And this monitoring is especially important in any strategy to lose weight.

Some doctors lower their patients' insulin or oral insulin-stimulating drugs the day they start on a weight-loss diet. This prevents a frightening episode of low blood sugar (hypoglycemia) four or five days into the diet (which happens if blood sugar drops and insulin or oral drug dosage is still high). Most successful at losing weight, with fewest hypoglycemic episodes, are diabetics who carefully monitor their blood sugar and consult with their doctor as often as every week about having their drug dosage lowered as their blood sugar drops.

Note: Diabetics whose fasting blood sugar is over 240 may need to lower their blood sugar first, then reduce their drug dosage. And for thin diabetics, the best treatment is drugs. Losing weight won't help.

Get smart about hypoglycemia. "I'm so attuned to my physical condition that when my blood sugar drops, and I feel 'fuzzy,' I still know exactly what to eat," says Charlene Postigo, a diabetic for five years. She consumes precisely what will bring her blood sugar back to normal—no more. That's 4 ounces of orange or apple juice or 4 to 6 ounces of milk. To make sure it's worked, she waits 20 minutes, then tests her blood sugar. Fear of falling into a diabetic coma leads even non-drug-dependent diabetics to overtreat low blood sugar with bowls of ice cream or peanut butter and jelly sandwiches. That only adds to their problems by piling on pounds. They need to learn how to raise their blood sugar without overeating.

Abide by the six-month rule. You've lost the weight. Now what? Well, for about six months, you've got to be very careful about what you eat because this is when you could easily regain those hard-to-shake pounds, diabetes nutritionists say. You'll be eating out, adding back desserts, maybe even having a drink once in a while. "Diabetics who do best realize the maintenance phase is tricky because it's a time when they could lose control," says Christine Beebe. "Those most successful at maintaining their weight loss get plenty of guidance and support during this period."

Go high-carb. Diabetics used to eat high-protein meals based on meat and laden with saturated fat. Bread, potatoes, and other starches were doled out in microscopic portions. Vegetables weren't bad, but they weren't considered helpful in lowering your blood sugar levels.

Based on research from the last ten years or so, those guidelines have been revised. Now the ADA recommends a high-fiber, high-complex-carbohydrate, low-fat diet. Why? For one thing, it's been found that the fibers in whole grains and some fruits and vegetables prolong sugar absorption, stabilizing blood sugar levels. Also, by shifting away from fats, especially saturated fats, the ADA is acknowledging that cardiovascular disease is a leading cause of death among diabetics.

And now it's also clear that complex carbohydrates (found mostly in whole grain products, beans, and vegetables) can be big pluses in any weight-loss plan. Since they're generally not calorie dense (few calories per unit of weight), you can eat a lot, satisfying your appetite without adding on extra pounds.

Keep it simple. The fewer changes you have to make in your diet, the easier it will be to follow. Forgo bean sprouts and seaweed in favor of broccoli and romaine if that's your preference. Reducing saturated fats from meats (using ground turkey instead of beef, for instance) and dairy products (using skim milk and lower-fat cheeses) may be all that's needed to get your diet in line. Most people have only two or three different breakfast and lunch menus and about ten dinner menus. They can work with these menus, adding whole grains or vegetables, subtracting fats and sugars, to make them healthier.

Making Workouts Work

Exercise also scores high in fighting Type II diabetes. "Exercise appears to help muscle cells take up and use sugar, even when there are lower levels of insulin in the blood," explains Gerald Reaven, M.D., a Stanford University professor of medicine and endocrinologist. That's crucially important because in Type II diabetes, insulin resistance (inability to use insulin properly) is a major concern.

Also, regular exercise can boost a sluggish metabolism to burn off more calories. That's why regular exercise can help people lose weight more easily, and, just as important, keep it off.

Walking is the activity most often recommended by doctors who treat diabetes. Why? Because the average Type II diabetic is 56 years old, overweight, and has been sedentary most of his or her life. Walking is the gentlest, most convenient way for these people to ease into activity and keep it up.

For More Information . . .

Want to know more about diabetes? The American Diabetes Association has cookbooks, nutritional guides, and other publications for anyone interested in good nutrition. Just out: Exchange Lists for Weight Management, a weight-loss program for people who are obese and suffer from diabetes, high blood pressure, or heart disease. With this program and your dietitian's help, you can plan a safe and effective diet. For more information, contact your local ADA chapter or affiliate, listed in the white pages of your phone book, or contact the Diabetes Information Service Center at (800) ADA–DISC. Residents of Virginia and metropolitan Washington, D.C., call (703) 549-1500.

Here are some strategies for making workouts as easy and effective as they can be.

Keep it steady and regular. Exercise seems to have a beneficial effect on blood sugar for up to 48 hours, so exercising faithfully at least every other day will produce the best results. If you take insulin or insulin-stimulating drugs, exercising the same time each day, for the same amount of time, can make it easier to control blood sugar.

Exercise an hour after meals. Exercise can sometimes lower blood-sugar levels too much, causing hypoglycemia. (This is more likely to occur if you use insulin.) But if you exercise about an hour or so after meals, when levels of blood sugar are peaking, hypoglycemia is less likely.

Check your feet. If you have diabetic nerve damage, you may not be able to feel if you have developed a blister. (If you're diabetic, even minor foot ailments may lead to serious problems if not attended to, like amputation of toes, feet, even limbs.) So visually check your feet every day. Look for red "hot spots," areas of early inflammation, cracks between the toes, and blisters. If irritation develops, don't delay seeing a doctor.

Wear running or walking shoes. Today's running and walking shoes do a super job of cushioning tender diabetic feet. (A study on running shoes showed they do a better job than street shoes at preventing blisters in diabetics. Some doctors tell their diabetics to wear nothing but running shoes.) Well-ventilated shoes (with mesh vents) and socks of synthetic fibers or cotton/synthetic blends that wick sweat away help prevent blisters, too.

Always carry identification. Use a tiny, strap-on wrist wallet or a fanny pack to carry your vital statistics. Include your name, the name of your doctor, the names of medications you're using currently—and the dosages—your address and telephone number and pertinent information about your medical condition.

Avoid head-low positions. If you're suffering from diabetic eye problems, avoid strenuous, head-low exercises like weight lifting or slant-board sit-ups, which can cause hemorrhaging and retinal detachment. Instead, go for walking, swimming, or cycling. These activities will help you shape up safely.

CHAPTER 13

Fighting Back against Chronic Fatigue

Tens of thousands of Americans may have "chronic fatigue syndrome," which causes fever, muscle aches, mental confusion, and more.

When Nannette Piscitelli's "flu" lasted almost two weeks during January 1986, she thought she was just run down. When she finally felt a little better, she went back to her job as a planner at a *Fortune* 500 company. Then in April, besides feeling overtired, she started getting headaches, lost her train of thought often, and had trouble walking. A brain scan found nothing wrong.

In August, a blood test revealed that she had high amounts of certain antibodies (proteins that fight foreign substances) in her blood. By then she was working only half days because of her constant fatigue and pain. The next month, she began having massive migraine headaches. "After a few more months, I didn't feel as much pain or weakness, but I was exhausted," she says. "I no longer was productive in my job. So I stopped."

Piscitelli's strange malady has been called the "yuppie flu," "Raggedy Ann syndrome," and bunk—but it's for real. It's chronic fatigue syndrome (CFS), an illness of continual dog-tiredness, achy muscles, fever, drowsiness, and the blahs that lasts months, even years. And tens of thousands of Americans may have it.

It doesn't hit just women, either. Anyone can be affected—from 30 percent to 40 percent of CFS victims are men, and others with the syndrome include children under age 10, teenagers, and men and women in their fifties and sixties. The disease strikes people in all socioeconomic groups, races, and walks of life, from all over the world.

But although scientists don't yet know exactly what causes CFS, there's new hope for dealing with it. Finally, after a lot of confusion about what CFS really is and even if it actually exists, medical experts are pinning it down and learning more about how to curb it. And they've put out the good word: CFS is not a fatal disease, and most people who suffer from it get better when they learn how to fight it.

Who Has It, Who Doesn't

About one in five people who walk into a doctor's office complain that fatigue is disrupting their lives. Yet only 3 to 5 percent fit the criteria of CFS devised by more than a dozen experts along with the Centers for Disease Control (CDC) in Atlanta and published in 1988.

According to these criteria, people who truly have CFS are those who've suffered a debilitating fatigue (or easy fatigability) that's lasted at least six months. They also must have ruled out (with their doctor's help) any other physical or psychiatric diseases that may mimic CFS symptoms, like acute nonviral infections, depression, hormonal disorders, drug abuse, or exposure to toxic agents. Then they must have at least 8 of the following 11 symptoms recurring or persisting for six months or more: chills or mild fever; a sore throat; painful or swollen lymph glands; unexplained general muscle weakness; muscle discomfort; fatigue for at least 24 hours after previously tolerated exercise; a headache unlike any previous pain; joint pain without joint swelling or redness; complaints of forgetfulness, excessive irritability, confusion, inability to concentrate, or depression; disturbed sleep; and quick onset of symptoms within a few hours or days.

Such symptoms are common to a variety of diseases, and chronic fatigue alone does not a CFS diagnosis make. So it's important to meet fully the CDC's criteria before your doctor can declare you a bona fide CFS victim. After all, some of us, because of our lifestyle, should be tired. A mother of three who gets only 4 hours of sleep each night is bound to be physically exhausted. Psychological stresses can also make you tired.

Besides having specific criteria for diagnosing CFS, scientists also know that many CFS sufferers have common traits. Some people with CFS often have several abnormal immune-system responses. Some, for example, have high levels of antibodies in their blood, normally a sign of the presence of bacterial or viral agents. CFS sufferers say that their fatigue started abruptly when they had a specific infection, such as the flu. They may even be able to name the exact day they took sick. The syndrome often begins during a stressful time, such as during a divorce, career change, or a death in the family. Also, many CFS people say they're depressed, but it isn't clear whether the depression caused CFS or developed later when "patients are sick and tired of being tired," says Stephen Strauss, M.D., chief of medical virology at the National Institute of Allergy and Infectious Diseases.

CFS sufferers also are more likely to have allergies, and their immune system may not produce the normal amount of chemicals that regulate the body's responses to disease.

In Search of a Cause

Over the years, doctors have come up with unproven and dubious explanations for the malaise: iron-poor blood (anemia), low blood sugar (hypoglycemia), environmental allergy (20th-century disease), or systemic yeast infection (candidiasis).

At one time, scientists considered Epstein-Barr virus (EBV) as a possible cause of CFS, since many—but not all—CFS sufferers have EBV in their blood. Some researchers believe that EBV may cause the syndrome in people who never recovered from mononucleosis. Others hypothesize that EBV or other viruses slumbering in the body somehow are reawakened to cause the symptoms. New evidence, however, indicates that EBV alone doesn't appear to be the culprit.

Most patients with CFS have features that overlap with the disorder called fibromyalgia, which is also associated with fatigue and muscle and joint pain. Some experts believe that CFS and fibromyalgia may actually be the same condition in many cases. If the two syndromes are the same, then the number of CFS patients may be enormous, since three to six million Americans have been diagnosed as having fibromyalgia.

To study CFS and to try to zero in on possible causes, the CDC has asked doctors in Atlanta, Grand Rapids, Reno, and Wichita to gather detailed information about the onset of CFS, what symptoms they see, and the course of the illness. "Some things point to a virus, but we are looking at everything—pesticides, fertilizers, varnishes, paints, household construction, and insect bites," says Walter J. Gunn, Ph.D, principal investigator of the CFS surveillance system at the CDC. "If we can get a solid group of patients who meet the case definition, eventually we may find some common cause."

Getting a Diagnosis

So if you believe you meet the CDC's criteria for chronic fatigue syndrome, you should be tested and have an adequate workup. Your family physician's office is probably the best place to start the investigation. With some simple tests, your doctor should be able to rule out other illnesses that may look like CFS. Such tests include autoimmune-disease tests, a complete blood count, endocrine-disease studies, liver and metabolic tests, a kidney screen, and a urinalysis.

Most people with CFS end up seeing several specialists to exclude other causes of the flulike symptoms. Nannette Piscitelli, for example, saw a rheumatologist, an orthopedist, a neurologist, and a psychiatrist before her family physician felt confident enough to make the diagnosis of chronic fatigue syndrome. University medical centers usually can provide all the consultants necessary to diagnose the syndrome.

Because it's not a simple disease to identify, some doctors are overdiagnosing the illness, leading patients who have not had appropriate workups to believe they have the syndrome. And some doctors who don't know exactly what CFS is are underdiagnosing it.

"Only about 50 percent of the people told that they have chronic fatigue syndrome actually have it according to the CDC criteria," says John Renner, M.D., a clinical professor of family medicine at the University of Missouri at Kansas City. He's seen the medical records of hundreds of patients diagnosed with the syndrome. "This is a complicated illness," he says. "First and foremost, it is something that takes a sophisticated medical workup, which includes immune studies (like blood work that looks at antibodies) and all the tests necessary to rule out other diseases. You want someone who understands the sciences of infectious diseases and immunology. If there's any doubt in your primary physician's mind, don't hesitate to consult an immunologist. And you probably will want to get a second opinion."

It's Not All in Your Head

One myth that CFS experts are trying to dispel is that the illness is all psychological. It's true that most people with CFS become depressed during their illness. But then so do most people with chronic illnesses. The question is whether they have a history of depression before the flulike symptoms appear.

When doctors treat fatigue as just a trivial psychological problem, they do CFS sufferers a disservice. The kind of fatigue they feel is serious and unrelenting. "I can drive to the grocery store and fill a lightweight plastic bag with food, and that's it for the day," Piscitelli says. "The quality of my life has been reduced tremendously. I can get people to buy groceries for me and to do my housework. But I can't get someone to help me concentrate or think clearly."

Many illnesses have gone through stages of skepticism only to become fully recognized, including multiple sclerosis, Legionnaires' disease, lupus, and AIDS. "Rather than saying that chronic fatigue syndrome is all in the patient's head, the skeptics need to listen to their patients more intently. The patients know their bodies and their emotions," says Orvalene Prewitt, a cofounder of the National Chronic Fatigue Syndrome Association, in Kansas City, Missouri. "We need to pursue all avenues to find an answer for this baffling flulike illness. Both the public and doctors need to know that there are people out there who really are sick."

Fighting Back

There's no proven cure yet for CFS, but there are treatments that often can help reduce the symptoms. And there's plenty of ongoing research to test new therapies. In part because of the symptomatic treatments, those who meet the CDC criteria usually do not get progressively worse, and many have gradually improved over time.

Most experts say that your best bet for treating symptoms is to:

- Get adequate amounts of rest. Measured doses of taking-it-easy do alleviate some symptoms.
- Eat right. CFS is not associated with vitamin or mineral deficiencies, but eating meals with adequate amounts of nutrients (including calories) does make a difference in how some CFS sufferers feel. Some report feeling better when the diet is low in sugar and fat.
- Do a small amount of exercise every day, even if it's just stretching. Chronic overexertion tends to worsen symptoms and may prolong the course of the disease. But most experts do not believe people will get better faster if they stay in bed. That can be psychologically and physically devastating.
- Ration your limited energy. "Every day, I think of energy credits," says Piscitelli. "The first credits I use are always for myself—I wash my hair, paint my nails. Then I balance out the rest over the day."
- If you are in a lot of pain, ask your doctor about pain medication.
- Get help to deal emotionally with the disease. You can seek counseling or get support from CFS patient groups (see "For More Information . . ." on the opposite page). "I went to a support group and found others like myself," says Piscitelli. "I also saw I needed some help on how to adjust to being chronically ill. After I had stopped working, I didn't call my friends to chat or get involved

in any activities. Now I've become the leader of the support group. Helping others helps me feel good."

Those patients who can maintain a positive attitude seem to cope the best. "I focus on living a balanced life and increasing my stamina," says Piscitelli. "Now I really appreciate the company of others. I'm not waiting to catch up with life. I do things in moderation, but I don't miss out on too much."

To help CFS sufferers, doctors have tried various drugs to help boost the immune system or to attack specific viruses. It's unclear, though, whether these medications can really help because they haven't been tested. One drug that was tested, the antiviral called acyclovir, was found ineffective.

But one type of drug—tricyclic antidepressants—appears, theoretically, to be designed specifically for this syndrome. "Depressive symptoms are part of the illness, but elevating depression is not the only reason to use antidepressants," says James F. Jones, M.D., of the National Jewish Center for Immunology and Respiratory Medicine, in Denver. "Tricyclic antidepressants have a number of pharmacological activities. They are potent antihistamines, which may help ameliorate allergies. They also are sedating, which can help patients get a good night's

For More Information . . .

To learn more about support for people with chronic fatigue syndrome, call the National Chronic Fatigue Syndrome Association at (913) 321-2278. Or write the association at 919 Scott Avenue, Kansas City, KS 66105. Include a self-addressed, stamped business-size envelope and 85 cents to cover handling fees. The association can give you the addresses and phone numbers of local chapters around the country, which offer information and support.

sleep. And they have anti-inflammatory effects." Dr. Jones has been able to relieve the symptoms of 70 percent of his CFS patients using one-tenth the dose of antidepressant generally prescribed to treat depression. He points out that antidepressants have not been evaluated in controlled trials of CFS patients.

Whatever treatment you try, CFS experts recommend that you beware of unproven therapies promoted as sure cures. The list of unsubstantiated therapies promoted as effective includes injections of hydrogen peroxide, homeopathic remedies, high colonics, and large doses of vitamin C or other food supplements.

"Until a cure is found, focus on safe, best-bet treatments," Dr. Renner says. "And remember that most people with CFS do learn to cope with it, and they usually get better."

CHAPTER 14

Take Control of Kidney Stones

Prevention is your best bet, and here's the diet that can keep you clean.

Just after his 27th birthday, Scott Davis was working at his computer when a sudden pain shot through the left side of his back, as if "something as big as a grapefruit was about to explode inside me." He'd been feeling perfectly fine, but all of a sudden there was this fearsome pain. After an agonizing night, he got up at dawn and drove himself to a local hospital.

X-rays revealed a couple of pebbles in Davis's left kidney, between the size of a pea and a marble. His urologist informed him that one way or another, these kidney stones would have to come out.

If Davis had developed the stones ten years ago or so, he would have faced two unpleasant choices: He could have let the stones pass one at a time and risked an ordeal of intense pain, or he could have undergone major surgery that would have required months for recovery. But Davis was very lucky. Thanks to medical advances, his urologist was able to offer a fast, painless treatment called extracorporeal shock wave lithotripsy (ESWL).

New Nonsurgical Treatment

In ESWL, the patient is lowered into a water bath, reclining on what looks like a massive 21st-century dentist's chair. During an hour-long procedure, a high-voltage generator sends up to 3,000 shock waves through the water and into the patient's flank. These waves demolish the stones while rippling harmlessly through the rest of the patient's body. The procedure runs about $7,000.

Despite the improvements in treating kidney stones, it's definitely preferable to avoid having them at all. Most first-time victims are young—between 20 and 30 years old—and otherwise in the best of health. Men are four times more likely than women to get kidney stones. The stones are rarely life-threatening, but the pain can make them feel they are.

What causes all the trouble are small, brittle, yellow or brown chunks of mineral salts that form in the kidneys or in the tubes that link the kidneys to the bladder. These renal calculi, as kidney stones are technically known, can be round, jagged, or branched. They may be as small as a speck of dirt or as big as a golf ball. Most are made up of either calcium oxalate, calcium phosphate, a combination of the two, or a variety of minerals and amino acids.

The Whys and Hows

Thousands of people can have the same amount of calcium in their urine, but only one or two will develop stones. Although a tendency toward kidney stones runs in families, environmental factors such as chronic dehydration may also cause them, as may a diet high in animal protein (associated with uric acid stones) or dairy foods (linked to calcium oxalate stones). Nobody really knows why men are more susceptible than women, but one theory holds that female hormones help prevent the crystals from forming.

Although kidney specialists may not know exactly why kidney stones form, they do understand how. The kidneys filter excess nutrients and impurities out of the blood and dump them into the urinary tract for excretion. If too much calcium winds up in the urine, calcium crystals begin to precipitate like little snowflakes, much the way a glass of water into which you shake a lot of salt "snows" salt crystals. But unlike little snowflakes, these crystals don't melt. In fact, they snowball, and their sharp edges wreak havoc.

"Extremely severe and sudden back pain is often the first sign of a kidney stone," says Jerome Kassirer, M.D., a New England Medical Center nephrologist. "But in men, a stone might also cause pain in the groin or testicle." Because of the pain's location, doctors occasionally mistake kidney stones for testicular trouble. An x-ray can usually distinguish the two.

"If the stone measures less than ½ centimeter in diameter—that's just under ¼ inch—there's an 80 percent chance the patient will pass it on his own," says C. Lee Jackson, M.D., a urologist at the Cleveland Clinic in Fort Lauderdale, Florida. "We prescribe pain medication and plenty of fluids, and we give the patient a strainer to collect the stone. If it doesn't pass after a month, we consider further treatment."

If you get kidney stones once, you run a 10 percent risk of developing more within a year and an 80 percent chance of developing a new stone within 30 years. Thiazides, a family of diuretics commonly used to treat high blood pressure, are often prescribed to prevent stones from recurring. Another drug, allopurinol, is sometimes prescribed to avert the formation of stones that contain calcium or uric acid. A new Japanese-made drug, marketed here under the name Thiola, has been found effective in controlling the formation of cystine stones.

A Preventive Diet

Since the foods you eat affect your body's ability to form kidney stones, doctors often recommend a change in eating habits to prevent recurrences, whether or not drugs are prescribed. Alan Wasserstein, M.D., director of the Stone Evaluation Center at the Hospital of the University of Pennsylvania, advocates drinking lots of water, eating less meat, cutting way back on salt, and keeping a lid on ice cream or cheese consumption. He also tells his patients to go easy on high-oxalate foods such as spinach, chocolate, tea, cola, rhubarb, parsley, peanuts, and citrus fruit. If the patient's stones contain uric acid, he calls for restrictions on alcohol, sardines, anchovies, herring, and organ meats such as liver. As additional insurance, Dr. Wasserstein often prescribes vitamin B_6 and magnesium supplements because they reduce oxalate levels and inhibit stone formation in some people. Conveniently, this low-fat, low-salt diet is as good for the heart as it is for the kidneys.

CHAPTER 15

Best-Bet Arthritis Centers

Find out which locations are considered the best in the country and what they can do for you.

One out of every seven of us can expect to battle arthritis in our lifetime. That means that one in seven of us will be looking for the best arthritis care we can find. The question is To find the best, where should we look?

The answer is, it depends. Arthritis comes in many forms and degrees. The best treatment for routine problems may be found in a few simple visits to your family physician or rheumatologist. Not-so-routine problems may demand a trip to a highly specialized center.

One thing is certain: You can be guaranteed the best care possible by contacting one of the arthritis centers designated to receive research funds from the National Institute of Arthritis and Musculoskeletal and Skin Diseases (NIAMS). A number of outstanding centers and clinics across the United States compete for these funds. Those chosen represent the paradigm of state-of-the-art care and treatment, says Julia Freeman, Ph.D., NIAMS centers' program director. To be judged leaders in their field, they must demonstrate the deepest commitment to most, if not all, of the following components.

Basic and clinical research. To qualify to become a NIAMS center, medical research must be of the highest quality. "When laboratory investigators work side by side with clinicians, knowledge can be rapidly translated into new treatments," says John B. Winfield, M.D., director of the University of North Carolina's arthritis center.

That can be of particular benefit to patients with difficult or serious conditions who may find treatments or diagnostic procedures here that are unavailable elsewhere. Past studies that NIAMS supported determined the causes of Lyme disease and gout, which in turn led to the development of effective treatments for those diseases.

Experts from multiple disciplines. One leading arthritis expert calls it one-stop shopping—and he's not talking about your local shopping mall. "The growing trend is to locate rheumatology, orthopedics, and rehabilitation under the same roof," says Roland Moskowitz, M.D., director of the Arthritis Division, Northeast Ohio Multipurpose Arthritis Center at Case Western Reserve University. "For state-of-the-art diagnosis and treatment, you no longer need to make ten visits to ten different experts." Then one physician, usually a rheumatologist, can synthesize all this expertise and design an individualized program.

Specialists who treat "nothing but." There's a lot to be said for seeing a doctor who's a leading expert in your particular ailment. While NIAMS centers generally treat all forms of arthritis, they tend to superspecialize in two or more areas. These departments perpetuate their expert status by attracting future leaders in the field.

Innovative education for physicians. Education programs address questions like: How can we convince students training to be general practitioners that rheumatology would be a valuable elective? And how can we help family doctors become more knowledgeable about rheumatology? One program trains patients to be teachers to help medical school students fine-tune their examination savvy.

After a typical arthritis examination, the patient evaluates the student's performance. Doctors-to-be learn what to look for, how to touch and what questions to ask.

Patient empowerment. Arthritis treatment often requires that you, the patient, make changes in your approach to everyday activities. The more willing and able you are to share in the responsibility, the more lasting relief you're likely to find.

One innovative program that promotes self-reliance is "Educize" at the Northwestern University Multipurpose Arthritis Center, in Chicago. "The session starts with a specially designed exercise class featuring light-impact aerobic dance routines," explains Frank R. Schmid, M.D., practicing physician and former rheumatology chief at Northwestern University Medical School. "What follows is a discussion period, where the class members and instructor share problem-solving strategies. Ultimately, patients learn to develop their own insights about the management of their disease."

Improved services for patients. Health-service staffs look at patterns of how patients use various services. One of their goals is to provide better service at lower cost.

When to Go to a NIAMS Center

Because early diagnosis and treatment can head off permanent damage to joints and tissues, the NIAMS centers encourage patients to seek treatment at the earliest onset of disease.

But because of their expertise and comprehensiveness, NIAMS centers tend to see mostly the most difficult and complex cases of arthritis. "Patients with difficult diagnoses or who demand complex treatments ought to be referred to a large center capable of providing multidisciplinary care," says Dr. Moscowitz. "If you need a total hip replacement, for example, you don't want to go to a place that does one a month. You want a surgeon who does them every day."

That may mean you have to travel. The initial visit can take anywhere from half a day to several weeks. (Biopsies and x-rays, for example, may require a stay of several

days.) Once you receive diagnosis and a treatment program is set, you may return home, where your primary
physician can follow through with your treatment.

In addition to the NIAMS centers, there are excellent
regional university centers, medical-school rheumatology
divisions, and nonuniversity major clinics across the country that may be more convenient to your home. Discuss
all options with your primary-care physician before you
travel any distance.

Routine Treatment Closer to Home

Not all situations warrant the cost of travel, hotel stay, and
time off from work that a visit to a faraway large center
incurs. Such a trip is only necessary in unusually difficult
cases. If your condition is routine, there's probably no need
to travel farther than your family doctor's office.

Many arthritic conditions fall in between routine and serious. (One example would be rheumatoid arthritis that
doesn't respond to standard therapy with anti-inflammatory analgesics like naproxen and ibuprofen.) At that point,
your family doctor may refer you to a board-certified rheumatologist. (If he doesn't, you may want to ask him about
it.)

In addition to medical school and three years of internal
medicine, rheumatologists spend at least two years focusing specifically on diseases that affect the musculoskeletal
system. It's their job to keep up on the latest innovations
in arthritis treatment. It's quite common for a rheumatologist to design a treatment plan your primary physician can
help you implement.

Although there are many excellent rheumatologists,
"there are also some physicians who are giving arthritis
treatments that are not approved by the mainstream,"
warns Naomi F. Rothfield, M.D., chief, Division of Rheumatic Diseases, University of Connecticut Health Center,
in Farmington.

The Arthritis Foundation, a nonprofit, volunteer organization that works closely with NIAMS, may also help
you locate physicians who specialize in treating arthritis.

Contact your local chapter (check the phone book) or write the national office at P.O. Box 19000, Atlanta, GA 30326.

New England

Boston University Arthritis Center
Evans Medical Group
80 East Concord Street
Boston, MA 02118
(617) 638-7460 for patient information

World-famous referral center for amyloidosis (a condition in which organs and tissues malfunction due to excessive blood protein accumulation). About 100 patients participate yearly in amyloidosis clinical trials. Another specialty: fibromyalgia syndrome (characterized by general muscle aches and tiredness). Latest research involves the use of photopheresis for rheumatoid arthritis. Waiting list: one to two weeks.

Division of Rheumatic Diseases, University of
   Connecticut Health Center School of Medicine
Farmington, CT 06032
(203) 679-2160 for physician referral; write for patient
   information

Specialties: lupus and related reproductive problems, scleroderma, Sjögren's syndrome, Raynaud's disease, and rheumatoid arthritis (RA). Currently developing tests to help predict the progression (and therefore aid in treatment) of diseases such as scleroderma, lupus, and Raynaud's. Promising new treatments: IV gamma globulins or cyclophosphamide (to stop antibody production) in lupus; methotrexate for RA. Waiting list: six weeks to two months.

Robert B. Brigham Arthritis Center
Brigham & Women's Hospital
75 Francis Street
Boston, MA 02115
(617) 732-5325 for patient information

Specialty: rheumatoid arthritis. Promising RA treatments under study: methotrexate, cyclosporine A, macrophage modulator, and interferon gamma. Pioneering research done here led to the FDA's approval of methotrexate, a new, potent drug that reduces pain and inflammation. Waiting list: two to four weeks.

Middle Atlantic

The Rheumatic Disease Clinic at the Hospital for Special Surgery
Cornell University
535 East Seventieth Street
New York, NY 10021
(212) 606-1328 for patient information

Specialties: lupus, vasculitis syndromes (a group of diseases that are marked by inflammation of the blood vessels), muscle disease, RA, and pediatric rheumatology. World-renowned orthopedic service, with leadership status regarding the development, refinement, and application of joint replacements. Research focuses on musculoskeletal disease. Waiting list: about two weeks.

South

Duke University Arthritis Center Clinic
Rheumatology Appointments
   Coordinator
Box 3809
Durham, NC 27710
(919) 684-3956 for patient information

Specialties: connective tissue diseases (lupus and Sjögren's syndrome), RA, osteoarthritis, vasculitis, Wegener's granulomatosis (a triad of sinusitis, inflammatory lung disease, and kidney inflammation). Receives special funding for RA research. Promising treatments: methotrexate for RA. Waiting list: one to three weeks.

UAB Arthritis Center
University of Alabama Medical Center
Russell Ambulatory Center
1813 Sixth Avenue
Birmingham, AL 35294
(205) 934-1443 for patient information

Specialties: comprehensive-care unit for various other forms of lupus, state-of-the-art joint replacement, patient education, and physical and occupational therapy. Promising treatments: clinical trials with experimental drug therapy. Waiting list: one day to two weeks.

University of North Carolina
Thurston Arthritis Research Center
932 FLOB, Room 231H, CB#7280
Chapel Hill, NC 27599
(919) 966-4191 for patient information

Specialties: lupus (particularly systemic lupus erythematosus) and other autoimmune diseases, occupationally induced rheumatology (carpal tunnel syndrome, for example), pediatric rheumatology. Promising treatments: joint replacement and clinical trials with experimental drug therapy. Waiting list: one day to several weeks.

University of Tennessee
Department of Medicine
956 Court Avenue, G326
Memphis, TN 38163
(901) 528-5737; ask for the clinical coordinator

Three separate clinics treat rheumatic disorders: Veterans Administration Medical Center in Memphis, Regional Medical Center in Memphis, and the University Physicians Foundation. Specialties: degenerative arthritis, gout, psoriatic arthritis, Reiter's syndrome, ankylosing spondylitis (arthritis of the spine), and pediatric arthritis. Receives special funding for RA research. Bonus: This is a multispecialty clinic. Patients with other medical problems can be referred within the clinic to a specialist in that area. Waiting list: Depends on particular specialist.

The University of Texas Southwestern Medical Center at
    Dallas
Division of Rheumatic Diseases
5323 Harry Hines Boulevard
Dallas, TX 75235–9060
Write for patient information

A NIAMS specialized research center for rheumatoid arthritis. The largest center doing ankylosing spondylitis research. Specialties: inflammatory arthritis conditions, particularly those affecting the spine, and lupus erythematosus. Promising treatments: Several new experimental treatments for systemic lupus erythematosus, RA, and scleroderma are available here and nowhere else. Waiting list: one to three weeks after doctor's referral.

Midwest

Department of Orthopedic Surgery
University of Minnesota
420 Delaware Street SE
Box 189
Minneapolis, MN 55455
(612) 625-1177 for patient information

A NIAMS specialized research center for osteoarthritis. Specialty: sports-related knee injuries and spine deformities that produce arthritis. Research investigation focuses primarily on identifying causes of osteoarthritis. Waiting list: two to six weeks (shorter for knee problems, longer for spine problems).

Indiana University Multipurpose Arthritis Center
541 Clinical Drive
Indianapolis, IN 46223
(317) 274-4225 for patient information

Specialties: arthritis in the elderly, particularly osteoarthritis, dermatomyositis/polymyositis, and amyloidosis. In addition to being a NIAMS multipurpose arthritis center, also designated one of three specialized centers of research in osteoarthritis. Its unique Performing Arts Medicine Clinic treats performance-related health problems in instrumentalists, vocalists, and dancers. Waiting list: varies according to patient need and specialist availability; may be as long as one month.

Northwestern Medical Faculty Foundation
222 East Superior Street
Chicago, IL 60611
(312) 908-8628 for patient information

Specialties at the adult division: autoimmune diseases like lupus and scleroderma, and RA. Has a comprehensive rehabilitation program. One-of-a-kind Educize program—modified aerobic dance exercises followed by group problem-solving discussion—enhances patient self-reliance.

Special pediatric arthritis division at:

Children's Memorial Hospital
2300 Children's Plaza
Chicago, IL 60614
(312) 880-4360 for information

Section of Rheumatology
Rush-Presbyterian/St. Luke's Medical Center
1725 West Harrison, Suite 1098
Chicago, IL 60612
(312) 942-8268; ask for the appointments coordinator

A NIAMS specialized research center for osteoarthritis. Also: Lyme disease center, osteoporosis center, joint-replacement program, sportsmedicine center, and back-pain program. Very active, new-drug clinical investigation program. People who are interested in volunteering for studies can contact the Arthritis Clinical Research Center at (312) 942-8799. Waiting list: one to two weeks.

University Hospitals Arthritis and Spine Center at Case
   Western Reserve University
2074 Abington Road
Cleveland, OH 44106
(216) 844-3168 for patient information

Specialties: osteoarthritis, lupus (specifically systemic lupus erythematosus), osteoporosis, total joint replacement, sportsmedicine. One of the few clinics in the country to specialize in the treatment of muscle disease. Internationally recognized spine center. Waiting list: two to three weeks.

University of Michigan Hospitals
Department of Internal Medicine
Division of Rheumatology
3918 Taubman Center
Ann Arbor, MI 48109–0352
(313) 936-5491 for information; (313) 936-5580 for
appointments

One of the oldest and largest arthritis centers in the world. Specialties include lupus, knee and foot problems, and gout. Promising new treatments include immunosuppressive therapies for autoimmune diseases. Waiting list: Patients can be accommodated quickly as need dictates.

Pacific
Rosalind Russell Arthritis Center
University of California Medical Center
400 Parnassus Avenue
San Francisco, CA 94143
(415) 476-1192 for patient information

Specialties: rheumatic diseases, RA, systemic lupus and allied diseases, osteoarthritis, and gout. Rheumatologists, orthopedists, and a physical therapist on staff. Waiting list: one day to two weeks.

Scripps Clinic and Research Foundation
Division of Rheumatology
10666 North Torrey Pines Road
La Jolla, CA 92037
(619) 554-8585 for patient information

Specialties include full spectrum of arthritis and rheumatic diseases: RA, systemic lupus erythematosus, polymyositis, dermatomyositis, and scleroderma. Special interest in Sjögren's, RA, lupus, and all forms of vasculitis, including Wegener's granulomatosis and giant cell arteritis. Treats chronic neck and low back pain. One of the world's finest sleep centers, treats the sleep disorders often associated with fibromyalgia. A large multispecialty clinic with close ties to departments of orthopedic surgery, endocrinology, and neurology and a chronic pain center. Promising treatments: testing new arthritis medications. Waiting list: about one week.

Stanford Immunology and Rheumatology Clinic
S-101 Stanford Medical Center
Stanford, CA 94305
(415) 723-6001 to schedule an appointment

A full-service clinic covering all aspects of care for rheumatological diseases. This includes consultation, acute care, and continuing care for chronic diseases. Promising treatments: total lymphoid irradiation for advanced RA and lupus nephritis. Waiting list: two to four weeks.

University of California School of Medicine
Department of Medicine Professional Group,
   Rheumatology
UCLA–CHS 47–139
10833 Le Conte Avenue
Los Angeles, CA 90024–1736
(213) 825-6452 for patient information; (213) 825-9711 for
   appointments

Specialties: lupus, vasculitis, RA, ankylosing spondylitis, scleroderma. Famous orthopedic group has pioneered designs for total hip and knee replacements. Opportunities to participate in studies evaluating treatments are available. Waiting list: one week to three months depending on specialist.

Note: These centers will try to see new patients in urgent situations as soon as possible. Most of the centers accept self-referrals but prefer that a primary physician make the initial contact.

CHAPTER 16

Take Charge of Choosing a Surgeon

You don't have to settle for the first name your doctor recommends. It's your life. Here's how to protect it.

Surgery is a medical treatment fraught with peril, but it is also as close as you can get on earth to real miracles. Surgery saves lives we would never believe could be saved; it repairs damage thought to be irreparable; it restores function where none existed anymore.

Miraculous cures and unavoidable deaths are opposite sides of the same surgical coin. If you need surgery, you must not flip that coin; you must carefully choose your best prospect for cure and not leave your fate to chance.

The choice of the wrong surgeon can cost you your life, your ability to function, or the needless loss of an organ.

To find a good surgeon you're going to have to take charge and ask a lot of questions. If you find that difficult, have someone do it for you. Your advocate should be someone you trust, a friend or relative who cares about you and will make the effort on your behalf. The important thing is not who does it but that there is somebody taking charge. Here's some advice.

1. Ask your primary-care physician. He undoubtedly has a great deal of experience working with and observing the surgeons in your community. For routine problems, you may well find an acceptable surgeon within your geographic area, although for complicated or more serious problems your search should not be so limited.

If your primary-care physician makes a recommendation, be sure to ask what that opinion is based on—friendship, geographic proximity, reputation, or some independent evaluation of competence. Does he know how many cases like yours the surgeon does each year? Does he know the surgeon's track record with the operation—his mortality rate and his complications rate? If he doesn't, will he find it out for you?

If not, then his recommendation is mostly anecdotal—based on those cases he himself knows about and the general reputation of the surgeon among his peers. That may be an accurate reflection of competence; it may not.

Ask your primary-care physician how well he knows the universe of surgeons practicing in the area. Is his experience based only on those who work at the same hospital as he does? Or only on those to whom he has personally referred patients? Or does he have a broader knowledge of what's going on in the community?

Get two names, not one, from your primary-care physician. Ask him to describe the relative strengths and weaknesses of each. This can enable you to see how candid and comprehensive his evaluation is. If he sees both his recommendations as equal and fully acceptable and can make no effective comparisons, then there is more cause to suspect the validity of the recommendation.

2. Get recommendations from other physicians. For major surgery, it is well worth seeking the advice of other physicians. In medicine, as in every other profession, those generally recognized by their colleagues as the superstars, the very best, are widely known and agreed on, particularly within the apex of the American health care system, the university-based hospitals. Ask a university-based specialist for the top ten cardiovascular surgeons or cardiovascular surgical centers in the country and the same names will show up again and again, no matter who is asked the question or which university he is affiliated with.

Within a given state or regional area, the same kind of informal consensus exists. Part of taking charge requires tapping into that information chain. How? By calling the nearest university center, asking to speak to the relevant department chairman, and then asking for his recommendation. If you feel uncomfortable doing this, ask your primary-care doctor to make the call for you. Just make sure he gets all the information you need.

- Who would be recommended if you could go anywhere, anywhere at all, to seek care? Why that person?
- Who would be recommended if you had to stay in your own state or region of the country? Why?
- If you live in a major metropolitan area with many top-flight medical institutions and practitioners, who would be recommended as the best person for your particular problem, and why?
- How does the regional person compare with the national recommendation? Is there anyone in your city or community he would recommend? How does that person compare with the other two?
- It is often useful to call the physician's first two recommendations directly, even if you can't get to them for treatment. If it's hard to see them, ask if they have personally trained doctors in whom they have confidence and who may now be practicing in your area—or at least in the same geographic proximity.

Ask the doctors this question: If they were sick themselves, where would they decide to go for surgery, and why?

By making these calls, you will be finding out who is thought to be excellent and why, and also, how the experts themselves would weigh differences in quality of care against convenience for your particular surgical problem.

You will be surprised at how many doctors will talk to patients who call them "out of the blue." If you explain why you are calling, quite often you can ask these questions yourself. The advantage of having your primary-care physician do it is that he may be able to give a more detailed summary of your medical condition and thus perhaps get better advice based on it.

3. Get recommendations from friends, relatives, and neighbors. In this area, a friend's advice has very real limitations. Having had similar surgery and survived without complications is not a qualification for judging the quality of the surgical care received.

Your friends can tell you some useful things, though. How well did the surgeon explain things? How much time did he spend answering questions before and after the surgery? Did he effectively communicate with family members immediately after completing the surgery? Was it easy to trust him, to have confidence in him? Did he take time for reassurance, for hand-holding, when needed? How did he react to requests for consultation and second opinions? Did he give a full report to the primary-care physician when responsibility for the medical care returned to him? Was the operation successful? Were there any complications? Any infections? How was the postoperative care?

The weight you give a friend's advice should be influenced by one other thing: How thorough was he during his selection process? If he followed the taking-charge approach, then he may have a lot of useful information to share with you, in addition to his impressions of the experience. So listen to your friends. Find out what their advice is based on. Weigh its significance accordingly.

4. Check the surgeon's professional qualifications. Is the surgeon specialty-board certified? If he is, in what specialty? How long has he been in practice, and how stable has his practice been? Surgeons who move from community to community, from state to state, may be doing so to escape the problems that they've left behind. Are they members of a university faculty, full- or part-time? Do they work in well-established groups or in solo practices? Who covers for them at night?

In general, you are looking for someone who is board certified and has a long and established track record with the procedure you will undergo. If a surgeon has just moved to his current practice, it is important to find out why. Most of the time the explanation is innocent enough, but every so often you will find someone who was not really moving into his new practice, but rather running away from his old one.

5. Check the hospital's record. Surgery is not a one-person show. The surgeon is the head of the surgical team, but each and every member of that team is essential to the outcome of your operation. In general, good surgeons and good teams go together. But not always. The best surgeon can be undermined by an inadequate surgical team. There can be dramatic variation in the hospital mortality rates for the same operation. In general, for complicated procedures, such as open-heart surgery, a hospital needs a sufficiently high volume of cases to keep the surgical team's skills finely honed. To put it bluntly: If they do too few, too many of their patients die.

Until very recently, the track record of a hospital was never talked about in polite company. Certainly it was not something you could easily find out. Nor did many people even think of considering it when selecting a surgeon.

Let's be clear about this: Failure to carefully consider a hospital's track record can cost you your life.

Every hospital keeps records and knows, or is in the position to know, how well it does and doesn't do for particular surgical procedures. But until recently, that information was kept in-house. For who would willingly go to a hospital known for an unacceptably high mortality rate for a given procedure? So the facts have generally not been voluntarily disclosed—until recently.

The practice is changing now because of pressure from Uncle Sam, who pays the bills under Medicare. The government is entitled to collect information on Medicare beneficiaries about such matters as what an institution's mortality rate is for any of 16 specified categories of health problems. And through the U.S. Health Care Financing Administration (HCFA), these data are published for all to see.

In some cases, the data can be misleading. Hospitals to whom higher-risk patients are sent may as a consequence have a less-favorable reported mortality rate. And remember—the information published by the HCFA deals only with Medicare cases, not with the total number of cases diagnosed and treated at that hospital. But in general, the publication of these data has been a real service and has provided information for us all.

So how do you get the data? Ask the hospital. If the hospital won't tell you, ask your primary doctor to try to get it. If that fails, you can get the Medicare data that exists for that hospital. To find out how to get that, call either the HCFA headquarters in Baltimore, Maryland, at (301) 966-6885, or the regional office of the HCFA nearest you.

The bottom line: Before you go under the knife, put the hospital's record under the microscope. If they won't tell you their track record, and if you can't find it out from the other sources, go somewhere else.

6. Check the surgeon's record and personality. As in the choice of any doctor, it is important to interview the surgeon before you submit yourself to him for treatment. The easiest way to find out how many similar operations a surgeon has done is to ask him. And while you're at it, ask him about his own record.

You may find it difficult to ask this of the person you may decide to trust your life to. You may feel you don't want his skills to be affected by a personal dislike or resentment of you. The truth is that good surgeons, with lots of experience and an excellent track record, don't mind the questions. Poor ones, with the highest mortality and complication rates, have that record because of their skill level, not their dislike of patients.

Although personality is less important here than technical skill, it's still a factor to be weighed. The recovery from surgery is aided by confidence in and comfort with your surgeon. You wouldn't want to trade technical competence for bedside manner, but when you take charge, you're more likely to find an individual who combines the two.

If you have done your job correctly, by the time you talk to the surgeon, you will have a pretty clear idea of his reputation, his credentials, the quality of the hospital he works at, and, perhaps, what other patients have thought of him. You're coming in to close the deal, to take the last step. Whether you take it alone or have your advocate help you, it's a step that must be taken if you are to maximize your chances of making the best choice.

CHAPTER 17

Superclinics: Where Medical Mysteries Are Solved

Up to two dozen experts investigate a single case at these seven multidisciplinary centers.

Some time ago, a 56-year-old Massachusetts woman we'll call Betty first noticed an ache in her right heel. "It throbbed no matter what shoes I wore," she recalls. Then, after a few months, the heel became numb. Betty consulted a physician, who recommended a test for thin bones. "The test indicated borderline osteoporosis, but I had a feeling it was more than that."

In time, the strange feelings began creeping up the back of her right leg. First pain, then a numbing paralysis encased her leg from heel to hip.

Concerned, Betty sought the advice of a neurologist. "He examined my leg, even stuck pins in it," she remembers. "But I couldn't feel a thing. The doctor admitted that I had a problem, but sent me away without treatment. He suggested that we just wait and observe it." Betty's leg only became weaker, however. "Eventually, I couldn't even carry a bag of groceries up the stairs. I became so unsteady that I had to hold onto the banister with both hands to keep from falling."

Finally, when the toes of her left foot began to get numb, and her legs were so weak that she was almost unable to walk, Betty made an appointment at the Lahey Clinic, located near Boston. She had heard quite a lot about it and felt sure that it was one of the nation's top multispecialty clinics.

She had a thorough physical that included blood tests and CAT scans. She was examined by a neurologist, a neurosurgeon, and when tests revealed lung abnormalities, a pulmonary specialist.

Betty's strange paralysis was discussed among two dozen physicians. Together, they ruled out all but the rarest disorders. "We knew there had to be a progressive abnormality affecting her nerve roots (the nerves at the base of the spine, which control the legs), because the roots themselves were enlarged," says Paul Gross, M.D., the neurologist who was in charge of Betty's case. "But we didn't know what it was.

"We wondered if the lung scars held a clue. Certain features about them made us suspect sarcoidosis, an inflammation that can affect the lungs. In rare cases, sarcoidosis can affect nerves in the spine."

Finding Elusive Answers

Dr. Gross and a team of specialists consisting of a neurosurgeon and a radiologist searched for answers. "We were determined to get to the bottom of this," Dr. Gross says. "Exploratory surgery, we agreed, was the only way to determine for sure whether sarcoidosis was the cause of Betty's strange paralysis."

Betty consented. "I was convinced that surgery was my best shot at a solution," she recalls. "After all, a whole group of doctors said so; it wasn't just one person's opinion."

Amazingly, Betty's case proved to be as perplexing on the operating table as it did at the clinic's conference table. On initial inspection, Betty's spinal cord looked normal; there was nothing to point to sarcoidosis. But before closing the incision, the neurosurgeon phoned Betty's neurologist, Dr. Gross, to report the findings—or, more precisely, the lack of findings. Dr. Gross, whose office was just upstairs, ran down to the operating room to have a look.

Dr. Gross didn't see anything unusual either. But after some additional probing, he and the neurosurgeon, Paul

Dernbach, M.D., uncovered a growth in the nerve roots at the lower end of Betty's spine. The tissue was removed for analysis. And, lo and behold, the biopsy report confirmed that Betty had sarcoidosis of the nerve root.

The inflammation probably began in her lungs, where it left telltale scars, the Lahey Clinic doctors theorize. From the lungs, it migrated to the nerves in her spine and was progressively destroying them. This condition, Dr. Gross explained, is very rare. "Certainly this was the first case that anyone at the Lahey Clinic had seen," he says.

Betty's story does have a happy ending. After the biopsy, she was put on an anti-inflammatory medication (prednisone), which halted the damage, allowing the nerves to regenerate. Her left foot is back to normal. Over time, doctors expect full feeling will return to her right leg, too. Best of all, Betty says she feels strong and energetic again.

Solving Medical Mysteries

Diagnosing strange symptoms like Betty's takes real detective work. Clues are gathered; alternatives are considered. And as every detective knows, persistence pays. Unfortunately, tracking down the answers can be a long and frustrating ordeal for the patient, involving endless rounds of visits to different doctors.

But Betty and thousands of other people have found answers under one roof, at one of the country's top-notch multispecialty "superclinics," where physicians cooperate to diagnose and treat the most difficult problems.

You've undoubtedly heard the names of some of these superclinics. The Mayo Clinic, in Rochester, Minnesota, and the Cleveland Clinic, in Ohio, are very well known. But you probably don't know what it is that makes these clinics unique among hospitals.

Superclinics offer the latest high-tech diagnostic tools and treatments. But unlike most hospitals, where independent doctors have "privileges" to admit and treat their own patients, superclinics have physicians on staff. For patients with baffling or multiple health problems, this can offer an advantage. Highly qualified specialists in a wide variety of fields work as a team, putting their heads together dozens of times a day to exchange opinions.

Checking In

From the moment a patient telephones one of the superclinics for an appointment, things happen differently from the way they do at a typical hospital.

At some clinics, like the Lahey Clinic, you do not need a physician's referral to make an appointment. You just place a call to the clinic's central appointment desk. Trained personnel will ask you a few questions to evaluate the nature of your medical condition and determine which specialists you need to see.

When you arrive at the clinic, you'll receive a computerized schedule of doctors' appointments and tests. At the Mayo Clinic, the computerized schedules in their brown envelopes are called "passports." "Everywhere you go you see patients carrying their little passports around with them," a Mayo administrator observes.

Your first appointment will be with your designated "primary doctor." If after examining you, the doctor recommends additional tests or consultations, the computer will incorporate them in a revised schedule. You'll see your primary doctor at least one more time, at the end of your visit. You are also encouraged to contact your primary physician with questions and concerns after you return home.

If a doctor sees the need, he or she can arrange an appointment with another specialist at the clinic, ideally within a few days.

"It's not uncommon for a patient to come in with one complaint, say a cardiovascular problem, then routine tests disclose other problems, like a spot on the lungs or perhaps something unusual with the urine. By the following day, the patient has had consultations with the cardiologist, the pulmonologist (lung specialist), the urologist and the hematologist," Lahey cardiologist Bruce Mirbach, M.D., explained. If there is a relationship between the different concerns—as there was in Betty's case, with her lungs and her spine—it's likely to be identified early.

The efficiency of this system is one reason these clinics are popular: It's one-stop shopping for quality medical care. For persons with multiple medical problems, it's possible to arrange appointments with specialists for different problems—say an internist for a general exam, a dermatologist for a skin problem, an ophthalmologist for an eye check, even a psychiatrist for counseling—all in one visit. The larger clinics offer as many as 50 specialties. Whether the patient has come in for a routine physical or to check out an inexplicable symptom, the process can be far less stressful than a series of visits to widely scattered doctors over a period of several months.

"A patient doesn't come today, then come back in a month carting around his x-rays and photocopies of his blood-test report," notes John Libertino, M.D., a kidney surgeon who heads Lahey's Division of Surgery. "There's one file, one folder; every specialist who sees a patient writes in the same file. It's very efficient and much more streamlined than any other place I've been."

Not every symptom can be explained or treated, Dr. Mirbach points out. "Sometimes, after our evaluation, the best we can do is offer a patient reassurance that nothing serious is wrong, that nothing's been missed and that they do not require surgery or medicines."

Cooperation, Not Competition

The success of these clinics in diagnosing complicated problems hinges on a critical factor: teamwork.

Superclinics like Lahey, Mayo, Cleveland, and others are really gigantic group practices. The physicians who work there are actually on the clinic's payroll; they are not permitted to take outside patients (unlike the usual hospital physician). "The self-interest has been taken away from the formula," notes Dr. Mirbach. "It's the quality of our work that counts, rather than quantity of patients. That's not to say this isn't the case in nonclinic situations. However, the major clinics strive for this ideal." As a result, cooperation has replaced competition among the physicians.

"It's like being on a baseball team. You work with the same people all the time; you're less prone to go off in a misguided direction," says Dr. Libertino. Ray Gifford, M.D., vice-chairman of the division of medicine at the Cleveland Clinic, concurs. "There's a spirit of cooperation and camaraderie that I really appreciate."

It's this teamwork—this constant dialogue between specialists in different disciplines—that benefits the patients most. Teamwork means, for example, that a nonsurgeon like Dr. Gross can routinely drop in on an operation, as he happened to do in Betty's case, which was the key to unlocking the secret of her paralysis.

At the Lahey Clinic, even the organization of the building encourages multidisciplinary problem solving. Specialties that interact frequently are grouped together. "It's no coincidence that nephrology is next to urology," says Dr. Libertino. "Similarly, the neurosurgery, neurology, and ophthalmology departments are located together. I've got a patient here today with microscopic blood in his urine; the nephrologist came from down the hall to look at his CAT scan, to discuss whether there's a tumor in his kidney."

Complex Problems Identified

An important draw of these clinics is their experience with rare diseases. "People often come to these large clinics as a last resort or because something unusual is wrong. That gives us vast experience in rare and difficult problems," says Dr. Gifford, who worked at the Mayo Clinic before taking his position at the Cleveland Clinic.

"Each of us has an interest in some rare disease," adds Dr. Gifford. "Mine is pheochromocytoma, a tumor of the adrenal gland that causes a rather severe and unusual type of hypertension. This is so rare that most physicians, including many internists and specialists in cardiology, would never see it in a lifetime. Because of my special interest—and my work at Mayo and the Cleveland Clinic—I personally have seen over 150 cases," says Dr. Gifford.

A Guarantee of Good Care

Ultimately, any medical institution is only as good as the physicians on staff. What's reassuring about the superclinics is that they have rigorous criteria for admitting staff, and stringent, ongoing peer review.

At the Mayo Clinic, for example, many new hires come from Mayo's Graduate School of Medicine, where they are in training for three to seven years. "We get a good, thorough look at them before we decide to invite them onto the staff," says Mayo staffer Mary Ellen Landwehr. At Lahey, Mayo, and Cleveland Clinic, physicians in clinical specialties must be board-certified or board-eligible (meaning they are in the process of getting board certification).

The selection process is different from many community hospitals, Lahey chief executive officer Robert Wise, M.D., points out. Often, physicians at community hospitals are independent practitioners who apply for hospital privileges, for which the review may not be very strict. "At Lahey, we seek out top physicians to come to our organization. And we exercise very rigid control over physicians who do come.

"Each candidate is interviewed by an interdisciplinary group of physicians. A surgical candidate, for example, will be interviewed and observed by a dozen physicians in internal medicine, radiology, and surgery."

Because the physicians in a clinic do work together so closely, patients can feel more confident that each physician maintains a standard of excellence. "We're able to monitor and control the activity of a physician in his or her office, as opposed to a traditional community hospital, or an individual practitioner, where there's no control whatsoever over how they practice medicine in their own office," says Dr. Wise.

Superclinics' Shortcomings

The physicians interviewed by *Prevention* agreed, however, that the large group-practice system does have its drawbacks. Some people feel that it isn't personal enough. "Patients are sent from one office to another, from one test

The Superclinics

An informal survey of physicians came up with this list of seven highly regarded group-practice medical institutions, with an approach to patient care like that described in the chapter. Most of the clinics listed below also have branch offices in the same state (or out of state).

Cleveland Clinic Foundation
9500 Euclid Avenue
Cleveland, OH 44195
(216) 444-2200 or toll-free (800) CCF–CARE
About 400 physicians. Physician's referral not necessary.

Lahey Clinic Medical Center
41 Mall Road, Box 541
Burlington, MA 01805
(617) 273-5100
Approximately 250 physicians. Physician's referral not necessary.

Lovelace Medical Center
5400 Gibson Boulevard SE
Albuquerque, NM 87108
(505) 262-7000
About 200 physicians. Physician's referral not necessary.

Mayo Clinic
Rochester, MN 55905
(507) 284-2511
Approximately 900 physicians. Patients can self-refer. (Mayo recently opened two additional group-practice clinics out of state, in Jacksonville, Florida, and Scottsdale, Arizona.)

Ochsner Clinic
1516 Jefferson Highway
New Orleans, LA 70121
(504) 838-4000
Approximately 316 physicians. Physician's referral not necessary.

Scott and White Clinic
2401 South Thirty-first Street
Temple, TX 76508
(817) 774-2111 or toll-free in Texas (800) 792-3710
More than 300 physicians. Physician's referral not necessary.

Scripps Clinic and Research Foundation
10666 North Torrey Pines Road
La Jolla, CA 92037
(800) 992-9962 in Southern California; or (619) 455-9100
326 physicians. Physician's referral not necessary.

to another. Although each patient is assigned a primary physician, he or she sees that physician only a few times over two or three days. It isn't like having a family physician that you see off and on all your life. We're aware of the problem, though, and we do our best to minimize it," notes Dr. Gifford.

Another problem: Like every other medical system, the clinics are overburdened and there can still be long waits to see the doctors. Sometimes, it can take up to a few months to get an appointment at the most popular clinics. Don't expect to be seen right away unless you're involved in a medical emergency. (Some of the clinics do offer a walk-in service.)

Keep in mind, too, if you visit an out-of-town clinic, you may have to stay in a hotel for up to a week to see all the specialists you'll need to consult.

A Better Way

Nonetheless, the doctors who are part of these organizations assert that this is the best way to diagnose the most difficult problems. "We believe that, in the long run, organizational medicine of this type is a better arrangement than the traditional fragmented systems we've seen surrounding community hospitals," says Dr. Wise.

"There are many outstanding hospitals and independent physicians in the Boston area," adds Dr. Wise. "But if I had a complicated problem that defied diagnosis, I'd check into the Lahey Clinic. Or if they couldn't see me for some reason, I'd call the Cleveland Clinic."

We asked other physicians where they would go if they had mysterious symptoms. Again, without exception, they said they'd head for a superclinic.

CHAPTER 18

The Politics
of Home Testing

The technology is in place for many home tests but the FDA is afraid to trust people with their own health care.

Your son Billy has a sore throat. He has no temperature, and it's probably just a virus, but you still worry that it could be strep throat, a bacterial infection with potentially serious complications. Rather than taking off from work and sitting for hours in a doctor's office to get Billy's throat swabbed and cultured, you go to your medicine chest for an inexpensive home strep test. Within minutes, you know whether or not Billy really needs to see a doctor or have a prescription ordered by phone.

The technology is already in place for home tests for strep throat; sexually transmitted diseases; urinary tract and vaginal infections; and vitamin, drug, and cholesterol levels. And manufacturers are ready to release them. But the tests aren't making it to market because the government is afraid to trust people with their own health care.

Although home diagnostic tests have won qualified approval from the medical community, and Food and Drug Administration (FDA) chairman Frank Young has spoken enthusiastically about the possibilities of such testing, in practice the watchdog agency has taken a cautious approach to approving tests for home use even when their effectiveness is strongly supported by laboratory studies. Perhaps bowing to pressure from physicians and others, the FDA now requires home diagnostic tests to be distributed through physicians for several years before they are released over the counter.

Pharmacists typically support over-the-counter home tests, but many physicians do not. Even the best tests, they say, are susceptible to misuse and misinterpretation by consumers, which render them useless or even dangerous. Many medical authorities contend that without instruction from a doctor and/or pharmacist, people might misinterpret test results, forgo treatment, or treat themselves improperly.

"Laypeople don't always understand the importance of following all the directions and not cutting corners," according to Dr. Paul Bachmer of Port Chester, New York, who has studied home tests for the College of American Pathologists. He says inaccuracies are quite possible if the chemicals involved are used incorrectly, stored improperly, or used after their expiration date.

"Laboratory tests are not an exact science," says Dr. Jerome Wilkenfeld, spokesperson for the College of American Pathologists. "Tests are always an extension of a physician's knowledge. In medical school, physicians are instructed never to depend solely on laboratory tests for diagnosis." He contends that a trained technician is better equipped to read diagnostic tests than the average consumer. He compares self-testing to trying to repair your own car. "You wouldn't try to fix your car yourself," he says. "You'd go to an expert."

Not all doctors agree. "You might not fix your own car yourself, but you should check your own oil," says Abraham Chaplan, president of Preventa-Pak, a company that manufactures home diagnostic tests for vitamin C and calcium levels and for digestive tract function. In 1987 the FDA pulled Preventa-Pak tests from retailer shelves. The tests are still sold in Canada, where Chaplan says regulators have a different attitude about home testing. The Canadian government ruled that since Preventa-Pak tests do not test for life-threatening diseases, a false negative reading would do little harm. Those who don't believe they are able to perform the tests properly, the government concluded, rarely buy them.

"In the United States, however, a diagnostic test cannot be released until 'the mythical Midwestern woman with a sixth grade education' can easily perform it," says Chaplan. Last year, the FDA turned down First Response, a home test for strep, because it may have been too complicated for some users. Marketed in Canada by Tambrands, the strep test uses monoclonal antibodies to detect the presence of the bacteria and claims to give "easy-to-read results in only 12 minutes." The user swabs the throat and executes seven steps in color-coded vials. A positive control is included that produces a blue dot when the test is properly performed. Two blue dots indicated a positive strep response.

Test directions are explicit about swabbing the throat and answer questions such as, "Why it is important to say Aahh?" Consumers helped write the test's instructions and 99 percent of those who tried it completed the test properly. Even so, the FDA denied approval in a preliminary hearing in August 1988 because the agency said the company had not gathered enough data from "consumers of differing education levels."

Tambrands spokesman Paul Konney says the company has encountered no direct opposition to the strep test from physicians in this country. "Physicians are sophisticated enough to see that this is no threat to their business," Konney says. "Doctors appreciate that home strep testing increases doctor visits and brings in patients who ordinarily would think they just had a cold."

Differing Opinions

However, others like Dr. Edward Kaplan, professor of Pediatrics at the University of Minnesota Medical School, isn't convinced that rapid strep testing is a good idea. Although the 95 percent specificity rate of the home test (the test is specific for strep and doesn't produce many false positives by identifying other bacteria) is as good as traditional in-office throat culture testing, Dr. Kaplan contends that recent studies show that some home tests miss as many as 38 percent of strep cases. However, none of the tests in those studies used the color detection method used in the Tambrands test. Also, the undetected bacteria were present in concentrations some say were not high enough to cause problems.

Other public health issues are at stake in the home diagnostic test controversy. Home testing for AIDS, for example, could have psychological ramifications for those who receive positive test results without the support of health care professionals. And if strep test sensitivity is a problem, as physicians like Dr. Kaplan contend, strep and even rheumatic fever could become more widespread. Certainly not every physician or pharmaceutical company is acting out of greed rather than concern for public safety. Nor are all the FDA requirements frivolous roadblocks. For example, the positive control, the blue dot in the First Response test, was an FDA requirement—and a good one.

However, by and large, consumers are being protected from themselves. In our increasingly educated, health-conscious society, that protection may not be necessary. Diabetics, for example, have been self-managing their potentially life-threatening condition for years using sophisticated self-testing for blood sugar (glucose). Many also self-inject insulin. Diabetic self-care is much more complicated than strep or cholesterol testing, but the FDA takes the former for granted and prohibits the latter.

The FDA's gatekeeping on home diagnostic tests may even be harmful to our health. For example, although more

Home Tests Available Now

While there is plenty of opposition to many home diagnostic tests, the movement toward self-testing is growing. Millions of North Americans now spend nearly half a billion dollars annually on devices that monitor blood sugar and blood pressure and tests that detect pregnancy, ovulation, and some types of cancer. Industry analysts expect sales of home medical tests to more than double in the next two years and quadruple to more than $3 billion by 1995. Private companies are developing over-the-counter home tests for allergies, strep throat, thyroid problems, and sexually transmitted diseases.

Here are today's five most popular self-tests.

Pregnancy. Seven to eight million women use home pregnancy tests. Accurate, fast, and convenient, these kits test urine for the presence of hormones indicating pregnancy. Dr. Sharon Dooley, a professor of obstetrics and gynecology at the Northeastern University Medical School says, "I think their quality is excellent." The tests cost $10 to $15 and can detect pregnancy as soon as one day after a missed period.

Ovulation. In 1986, 500,000 home ovulation tests were sold, mostly to women trying to become pregnant. The test predicts ovulation by testing for a sudden surge in the concentration of luteinizing hormone in the urine. Ovulation takes place within one day of such a surge. Women must test their urine each morning for six to nine days. Older tests, which boasted 90 percent accuracy, took more than 30 minutes. Newer tests are faster, but their accuracy is still in question. Ovulation tests cost $17 to $25 and should not be used as a method of contraception.

Blood pressure monitors. Hypertension authority Dr. Edward D. Frohlich of New Orleans says blood pressure monitors are "very useful." They allow people with hypertension to monitor their blood pressure regularly so drug treatment and self-care measures can be adjusted. Blood pressure monitors, which range from $22 to $150, come in two models: one that requires a stethoscope and one with a digital display that does not. The American Heart Association contends that digital models are more sensitive to noisy body movements, or movement of the device, which can interfere with accurate readings. Dr. Frohlich recommends buying machines that can be calibrated by hooking up to a physician's mercury column instrument or otherwise periodically adjusted.

Blood glucose. More than one million people with diabetes depend on daily self-monitoring of blood glucose. In some, a tiny lancet is used to prick the finger; the sugar in a drop of blood causes a chemical reaction on the test strip. Others require small, battery-powered meters. Although blood glucose self-tests are not as accurate as laboratory testing, home testing allows both diabetics and their doctors to make better informed therapy decisions. Diabetics often spend more than $750 annually on testing, depending on how often they test and which type of test they use.

Colorectal cancer. Former President Reagan's operation for colon cancer focused attention on the nation's number two cancer killer (after lung). However, researchers disagree about the advisability of routine occult blood testing. The American Cancer Society recommends professional occult blood tests periodically after age 50 but expresses concern that home tests produce too many false positives and false negatives. The test, which costs about $9, measures traces of blood in the stool that may indicate hidden tumors.

Write On!

In addition to writing to your elected representatives, you should contact the following:

Frank E. Young, M.D.
Commissioner, Food and Drug Administration
5600 Fishers Lane
Rockville, MD 20857

Surgeon General of the Public Health Service
200 Independence Avenue, SW
Washington, DC 20201

Louis W. Sullivan, M.D.
Director, Health and Human Services
200 Independence Avenue, SW
Washington, DC 20201

Office of Technology Assessment
Health and Life Sciences Division
600 Pennsylvania Avenue, SE
Washington, DC 20510

Senators Edward M. Kennedy, Orrin B. Hatch, Charles Grausley, and Claiborne E. Pell all serve on the committee that oversees the Office of Technology Assessment, and letters should be addressed to each senator.

than 140,000 North Americans develop colorectal cancer every year, many health experts do not recommend the simple screening test for occult blood. Some authorities contend such screening is useless because the tiny amount of blood the test detects can be caused by a variety of factors such as aspirin, hemorrhoids, bleeding ulcers, and even eating red meat. The tests, they say, can cause an unacceptably high proportion of false positives. For the blood stool test and other tests, consumer education and proper labeling may be a simple—and lifesaving—solution.

The FDA prevents us from learning things about our health we have every right to know. Our voices, consumer voices, haven't been heard. If you're concerned about this issue, let your representatives know.

CHAPTER 19

The High Costs
of High-Tech

*Between 1981 and 1988, the number of liver trans-
plants alone increased nearly 65-fold. Can our financial
metabolism survive the strain?*

When Bruce and Patty Miller's baby arrived prematurely,
both the newborn and the family's health maintenance
organization almost went under.

The Willow City, North Dakota, couple's baby spent his
first five months in intensive care surrounded by respira-
tors, oxygen concentrators, electronic breathing monitors,
and other high-tech miracle workers. Finally he began to
thrive; he's now a bouncing three-year-old. But the couple's HMO at the time, Heart of America of Rugby, North
Dakota, was bled nearly dry by the $300,000 bill he ran up
at a regional hospital.

"It took us more than two years to recover," says Cindy
Schwab, the HMO's operations manager. "We're keeping
our fingers crossed" that similar cases don't occur.

Heart of America's problem is at the heart of one of
America's biggest problems—how to pay for the medical

miracles that technology offers. In theory, we all embrace the new technology; after all, if a child will die without a liver transplant, the child *must* have the operation. But the issue becomes thorny when we ask who will pay for the transplant. Insurance companies are balking. Employers squeezed by rising health care costs are, in turn, squeezing employees to assume more of them. And employees are outraged.

"It's becoming much more evident that we will have to make ultimate decisions about our health care priorities," says Daniel Callahan, director of the Hastings Center, a think tank that studies medical issues. That probably means some form of rationing.

A Monster's Broken Back

It's hard to believe that it was only a few years ago that Margaret Heckler, then health and human services secretary, declared that the Reagan administration had "broken the back of the health care inflation monster." In that year—1984—the rise in the national medical bill was the lowest in decades, because of slowing inflation and cost-cutting measures.

But by 1986 the monster was healed, and health care spending was soaring. In 1987, the latest year for which figures are available, the U.S. health care tab rose 9.8 percent to $500.3 billion, or about 11.1 percent of the gross national product (GNP).

The monster can thank high-tech medicine for its restored health. New imaging systems, balloons to ream coronary arteries, genetically engineered drugs, and devices that zap cancer cells with heat—all are just what the doctor ordered for the ailing beast. By 1993, it is expected to devour 12.5 percent of the GNP; by 2000, a whopping 15 percent.

That isn't necessarily bad. Britain spends only about half as much per capita on health care as the United States does, but its citizens often spend years on waiting lists for high-tech palliatives Americans get for the asking. In Britain, patients sometimes have to wait years to receive artificial hips; every step during the wait causes excruciating pain.

Fat and Unhealthy

The U.S. system, though, has grown fat and unhealthy on its rich diet of high-tech goodies. Studies during the past few years indicate a fourth or more of our health dollars go for unneeded or questionable tests and treatments. The Blue Cross and Blue Shield Association estimates $6 billion to $18 billion is wasted annually on tests alone. Meanwhile, some 37 million Americans don't have health insurance and struggle to get even minimal care.

"If we knew we were getting value out of what we pay for health care, there wouldn't be as much concern about spending so much," says Joel Miller, head of medical practice research for the Health Insurance Association of America, a trade group in Washington, D.C.

Only about 15 to 25 percent of U.S. health care dollars are spent directly on medical devices and technology-related services. But indirect costs are much higher—at least half of the growth in the nation's medical expenses stems from new technology, medical economists estimate.

By enabling novel procedures, technology "provides new excuses for treatment," says Sheldon Greenfield, who studies health care issues at Boston's New England Medical Center.

For instance, machines that can temporarily take over the heart's blood-pumping duties opened the door in the mid-1970s for surgeons to perform coronary bypass operations. That, in turn, filled hospital beds with a steady stream of heart patients and generated countless bills for tests and treatment before and after operations. By 1982 bypass surgery accounted for about 1 percent of U.S. health costs, or $3 billion; now the bypass bill is more than twice that.

Although the laying on of hands is being replaced by the reading out of data in medicine, the great majority of physicians want to do what is best for patients. But technology tends to bring less pure motives into play. In competition for patients, specialists must buy the latest equipment. Then they have to use the devices constantly to pay for them. Dubious tests and treatments often follow.

Justifying the Costs

Similarly, doctors conducting research at big teaching hospitals with expensive machines must keep them in constant use to justify their costs, says a Boston medical researcher. His city, known for its three medical schools and a wealth of prestigious hospitals, is also known for its physicians' costly style of practice—some doctors refer to patients who died after a plethora of heroic, high-tech measures as having suffered "the Boston death."

For their part, doctors say the threat of malpractice lawsuits causes excessive use of medical technology. "Ninety percent of the time a good diagnosis of pancreatic cancer can be made from a good physical and history" of a patient, says Dr. Folkert Belzer, chairman of surgery at the University of Wisconsin medical school. Yet doctors usually order computerized x-rays called CT scans or even more expensive magnetic resonance image (MRI) scans for such patients, running up hundreds of dollars of bills for redundant information. "If you ever go to court, the experts [hired by a suing patient] will say the scans were needed," says Dr. Belzer.

Moreover, say doctors, patients pressure physicians to administer the latest technology fix and sometimes go "doctor shopping" until they get it. "In my parents' bridge club, it's considered a badge of honor to have had a cardiac catheterization," a procedure for treating clogged heart arteries, says Dr. John R. Ball, executive vice-president of the American College of Physicians. Dr. Kitt Shaffer, a Boston radiologist, says a patient recently called her seeking an examination with a "special hernia scanner," a device that hasn't been invented—yet.

Marketing Battle

Competition among hospitals also feeds the health care inflation monster. In Columbia, Missouri, a college town of 65,000, seven hospitals are vying for patients, including two general hospitals and the University of Missouri's medical center. Three of them have acquired MRI scanners, machines costing about $1.5 million apiece. Two hospitals are fully equipped for open-heart surgeries. In its television commercials, Columbia's Boone Hospital Center features its cutting-edge technology, showing, for example, its surgical "laser suites."

This year Boone raised the high-tech ante by investing in a $1 million upgrade for its MRI machine. The university hospital answered with an ace—it recently performed the area's first heart transplant. Still, "we do more open hearts than they do," asserts a Boone spokeswoman.

Besides attracting patients, high-tech offerings often yield spectacular per capita billings. A liver transplant can cost $250,000 or more, and several U.S. children have had four of them. A premature baby can run up bills of $500,000 or more. As for "the Boston death," don't ask.

Some doctors argue that the high-tech medicine they dispense saves money by replacing costlier alternatives. But a study by University of Pennsylvania researchers casts doubt on that. It showed doctors often continue to use old diagnostic tests after new ones are available. Apparently, says John Eisenberg, one of the researchers, doctors use both old and new tests on the same patients in hopes one test will catch problems the other one misses. Thus medical technology tends to "accrete" in hospitals, "increasing the cost of medical care," the researchers wrote.

Even when cheaper new technologies supplant old ones, the improvements typically open the door to treating more patients, pushing up total costs. In surgery, better ways to control infection, fiberoptic tubes for peering into the body, and other advances mean that "surgeons can now intervene for almost any purpose without [endangering patients]," says Dr. John Wennberg, an epidemiologist at Dartmouth Medical School in Hanover, New Hampshire.

Eight years ago, for example, transplanting a liver was a high-risk medical experiment. Now it's a fairly routine procedure—even 70-year-olds are getting new livers. Moreover, the number of potential liver donors is huge because the organ is the only one that doesn't deteriorate much with age. In 1988 there were 1,680 liver transplants in the United States, compared with 26 in 1981.

Most of the nation's high-tech medical bill, however, springs from more common treatments. In 1988 researchers studying the federal Medicare system examined 35 new technologies and found that just two of them would account for 38 percent of Medicare's 1989 cost increases: drugs to clear blocked arteries and coronary angioplasty, the reaming of clogged blood vessels with balloons snaked in through arteries.

While the Food and Drug Administration requires that new drugs be both safe and effective, there is no such regulatory oversight of medical procedures. Thus unneeded—and occasionally downright dangerous—high-tech treatments can proliferate without hard questions being asked about them.

In a study on coronary bypass operations, for example, researchers found that only 56 percent of the operations were clearly appropriate. Such findings are multiplying as health-care organizations put high-tech medicine under the microscope. Eventually, these "outcome" studies may reduce costs. For instance, when patients considering elective surgery know all the risks and benefits, they "tend to be more risk-averse than surgeons and often will choose to live with" an ailment rather than go under the knife, says Dartmouth's Dr. Wennberg.

Meanwhile, many hospitals are trimming health care fat by sharing some resources and eliminating others. Boston's Massachusetts General Hospital and New England Medical Center jointly purchased a $1 million lithotripsy machine.

But even if all the fat were eliminated, high-tech medicine might still overwhelm our ability to pay. "The amount of waste to be squeezed is finite," says William Schwartz, a health care expert at Tufts University. "But our stream of new technologies is like an open faucet."

Ultimately, says Dr. Ball of the American College of Physicians, beating the health care inflation monster will probably require "making certain assumptions about the value of saving a life." At the abstract policy level, that's hard enough. In specific cases, it will be even harder. "When it gets down to a treatment that has a 1-in-100,000 chance of saving a patient's life," says Dr. Ball, "the patient usually will say, 'I want it.' "

CHAPTER 20

Good-Bye to the Bedside Manner

By David E. Rogers, M.D.

Is the doctor/patient bond disappearing? This physician, trained in the 1940s, thinks so.

When faced with a sick patient suffering from an unknown ailment, is today's young physician less skilled than his predecessors in using his senses of sight, touch, hearing, and smell in arriving at an accurate diagnosis?

Absolutely.

Is he or she more often wrong because of the loss of those skills?

No. The diagnostic batting average is probably higher than at any time in the past.

Has the replacement of bedside diagnoses by technological diagnoses changed medicine?

Profoundly—and perhaps not always for the better.

Until recently, physicians were obsessed with diagnostic skills. Listen to doctors talk in the coffee shop or the cloakroom, and more often than not the conversation revolved around legendary calls made by great physicians on the basis of bedside observations. The thermometer, the stethoscope, the ophthalmoscope—all were technical advances that served to extend the physician's senses; they were cheap and portable and used personally by the physician at the bedside.

All of us who became doctors during the 1940s and before struggled to perfect such diagnostic skills. A good clinician could detect the smell of uremia, a diphtheritic throat, or diabetic acidosis on entering the room. The facial appearance of a patient with myasthenia gravis or Parkinsonism often permitted a quick call. The feel of the skin could suggest hyperthyroidism; the ankle jerk, myxedema. These were the daily fare of clinical bedside medicine.

As neophytes, we focused on the bedside skills of senior physicians. Years of practice made one better at this sort of thing, and we were determined to acquire those skills as swiftly as possible.

But now a series of miraculous new technologies has rendered such meticulous, physician-intensive observations obsolete—or so it seems to many. The CAT scan, magnetic nuclear resonance pictures, echocardiograms, sonograms, and the like can all produce detailed anatomic displays of what previously lay hidden in the head, chest, or abdomen. Almost without laying a hand on a patient, a physician can obtain startlingly accurate information about where things have gone wrong inside the human body.

A Sad Reality

Is that bad? Of course not. The diagnostic advances, and the positive things we can now do for sick patients when we know what is wrong, are breathtaking.

Why then does the atrophy of these bedside skills so sadden some of us? Is it just an exercise in nostalgia—like bemoaning the disappearance of the horse and buggy?

No, for several reasons. First, and most obvious, when the chips are down—in the home the small-town office—those bedside diagnostic skills still pay off handsomely. They can be the difference between life and death for many patients.

Second, these new technologies are frighteningly expensive. Substituting a CAT scan for careful history is part (though only part) of what is raising medical costs at rates

that so worry Americans today. Discriminating and re-
strained use of technologies would slow that rise.

But there are other, more subtle reasons to worry.
Clearly, the amount of "hands-on" physician time with
patients has been sharply reduced. No one can quantify
the precious bonding between physician and patient that
begins during the touching-feeling-looking-smelling process, but I tend to feel that it was—and still is—vital.

Yet too often these days I see young physicians fail to
really examine a chest carefully; instead, they simply send
patients down for an x-ray or a CAT scan. Those precious
moments in which the physician is talking to, examining,
and spending time with the patient are lost. And the emotional moat that separates patient and physician is widened.

Technology also seems to have robbed teaching of much
of its former joy—and benefit. The new technologies are
an enormous equalizer, and they tend to negate clinical
experience. Thus the youngest resident with a CAT scan
in hand may know more about the patient than I do—
even after I finish my evaluation. Part of that is wonderful.
For a young physician to know immediately what it took
me many years to learn how to detect is a medical advance
of the first order.

But again, there is a dark side. Residents may know
by virtue of technology what is physically wrong with a
patient, but they consequently tend to miss the personal
interactions I use with patients to try to make them feel
more comfortable and less fearful. Why do I sit on the side
of the bed of some patients? How is my listening different
from theirs? Why do I respond to a patient's questions,
worries, hopes, or fears in the particular way that I do?

Residents are so preoccupied with the problem of disease
that they fail to think much about the patient who *has* the
disease. And they forget (or never learn) how often the doctor himself must become part of the treatment, and that in
so doing, the doctor can often improve patient outcomes.

Physicians, I'm afraid, are losing something more than
they realize in letting those skills atrophy, and medicine
and our relationships with those who are sick are probably
poorer for it.

CHAPTER 21

Diagnosis
in the Fast Lane

There's no doubt they're quick—the question is, are they necessary?

In the old days of medicine—before the mid-1980s—patients visiting doctors would often have to wait a day or more for lab reports on blood samples or tissue cultures. Individuals needing more involved tests—like a stress electrocardiogram, with its treadmill, monitor, and related gear—would be bundled off to a hospital.

But that was before instant diagnostics.

Chemical analyzers and sophisticated scanning devices that once were found only in labs or hospitals now sit in doctors' offices, providing results for as many as 100 tests in a single hour. Studies estimate that 90 percent of primary-care physicians now perform tests in their offices—at an annual cost of more than $5 billion to insurers, employers, and patients.

In many respects, the change has benefited medicine. Patients, for instance, no longer face anxious intervals between initial office visits and final lab reports. Primary-care physicians, meanwhile, can identify and treat more problems on the spot, meaning fewer patient visits to specialists, labs, and hospitals. "A good, early diagnosis cuts down on exploratory surgery and expensive screening procedures," says Jerome G. Donahue, president and chief executive officer of Imex Medical Systems, Inc., a maker of diagnostic devices in Golden, Colorado.

Now the Bad News

But instant diagnostics can be a double-edged sword. The new tools in doctors' offices are also a new source of income. Insurers and third-party payers, as well as some physicians, say more doctors are now ordering excessive numbers of tests simply to pad their wallets.

"Tests are being done that have no relation to the illness," says Dr. Edward R. Pinckney, a former editor of the *Journal of the American Medical Association* and an internist in Beverly Hills, California. "Doctors are making less these days, so they try to do as many services as possible. Money is at the root of it all."

Physicians, of course, deny that they test for profit. But they concede that office tests are becoming an increasingly important part of their business.

That's partly because of advances in technology. Makers of medical equipment and tests are pumping out ever simpler, faster, and cheaper methods of diagnosing patients' ills. Until recently, test results on sexually transmitted diseases like herpes might have taken as long as three days to reach a physician. Now the test can be done in a doctor's office in 30 minutes.

Similarly, Henry M. Weinert, president of Boston Biomedical Consultants, Inc., a consulting firm, says that "before 1984 or 1985, basic chemical tests on liver and kidney functions had to be performed on instruments costing between $50,000 and $250,000, operated by a certified lab technician. Now the same machines sell for between $5,000 and $10,000 and can be operated by the doctor or a nurse." In the last several years, says Weinert, physicians have purchased about 40,000 such analyzers for their offices.

Patients' Expectations

At the same time that technology is *providing* more tests, patients are *demanding* more tests. "It's the expectation that goes with medicine now," says Dr. Nancy W. Dickey, a family physician in Richmond, Texas, and a trustee of the American Medical Association (AMA). "Patients want tests; they want something to confirm my diagnosis."

High on the current hit parade are instant tests for cholesterol. "It costs a doctor between 50 cents and $2 for a cholesterol test," says one supplier. "But they charge $5 or $15 or $50, depending on what they can get reimbursed."

Physicians' concerns about malpractice have also contributed to the growth of diagnostic tests. "I might be comfortable with a diagnosis," says Dr. Dickey, "but it might not hold up in a courtroom without something in black and white to back it up." In a Gallup poll commissioned earlier this year by the AMA, 75 percent of surveyed doctors said the threat of lawsuits has prompted them to order lab tests that aren't otherwise needed.

Beyond legal battles, however, increasing competition among doctors themselves has led to a greater reliance on office tests. If physicians don't offer on-the-spot lab reports or the latest devices that help diagnose, say, vascular disease, they risk losing patients, says Donahue at Imex. "There are too many doctors out there," he says, "and they're fighting for their lives."

Pressure Leads to Fraud

In some cases, the pressure to retain patients—and income—leads to outright fraud. In 1986, Northwestern National Life Insurance Co. in Minneapolis denied $275,000 in claims as fraudulent. Thirty-five percent of the total was attributed to unsupported testing and physician fees. In 1988, the company rejected $934,000 in claims; 94 percent were for unsupported testing.

"In the early days of fraud detection, doctors charged for tests they never did," says Rick Naymark, a spokesman at Northwestern. "Now they're charging for tests that aren't necessary."

To help fight the problem, insurers and doctors have started to publish guidelines for physicians that recommend when selected tests should be used. Blue Cross and Blue Shield, in conjunction with the American College of Physicians, has set standards for the 15 most common categories of diagnostic tests, among them x-rays and blood tests. The College of Physicians, for instance, recommends that extensive biochemical tests "not be done routinely" in annual physicals.

"Ethically, there's always a concern that doctors may run more tests because the equipment is there," says Dr. Dickey. "But it's not being swept under the rug. We're aware of the concern. That awareness will increase physicians' sensitivity and decrease the likelihood of abuse."

CHAPTER 22

How the Stress Experts Deal with Theirs

By Michael Castleman

Stress-management authorities lead lives as stressful as yours. Three experts reveal how they beat burnout.

Have you ever wondered how the stress experts deal with the curveballs life inevitably throws them? Do they simply sing verses from the Grammy Award–winning song by Bobby McFerrin, "Don't Worry, Be Happy"? Or do they keep some stress-survival secrets hidden away from us consumer types so they could always appear mellow, even when things weren't exactly hunky-dory in the stress-management trade. I had to find out.

My first appointment took me to the Harold Brunn Institute at Mt. Zion Hospital in San Francisco, where for more than 30 years, cardiologist Meyer Friedman, M.D., has been the director of cardiology research. Friedman, a grandfatherly physician with a soft voice and a warm smile, is the nation's elder statesman of stress management. Along with colleague Ray Rosenman, M.D., he coined the term "Type-A behavior," the hard-driving, hostile, time-pressured lifestyle that leads to substantially increased risk of heart attack.

During the late 1950s Dr. Friedman and Dr. Rosenman became frustrated by the fact that the accepted risk factors for heart disease—family history, smoking, obesity, high-fat diet, high serum cholesterol, and chronic high blood pressure (hypertension)—did not adequately explain the heart attacks many of their patients were suffering. At the time, the two researchers were trying to figure out why the socially prominent members of the San Francisco Junior League experienced significantly fewer heart attacks than their executive husbands. Black and European women suffered the same rates of heart attack as *their* husbands. What protected the Junior Leaguers? Dr. Friedman and Dr. Rosenman guessed diet, and launched a survey of the eating habits of 46 Junior League women and their spouses. During the study, Dr. Friedman happened to mention his quest for the elusive risk factor to one of the Junior Leaguers, who immediately said, "I'll tell you what's giving our husbands heart attacks. Stress, that's what."

Something clicked. Dr. Friedman thought about his patients, high-strung go-getters with perpetually furrowed brows who made coiled springs look relaxed. Then he remembered an incident from years earlier. An upholsterer had remarked how odd it was that in Dr. Friedman's waiting room, only the front edges of the chairs showed any wear. That observation had made no sense to Dr. Friedman at the time, but now suddenly it fit in. People who had heart attacks sat on the edges of their seats. They were like runners straining at the starting blocks, except the race never ended. They ran and ran and kept running—until finally their heart gave out.

Dr. Friedman and Dr. Rosenman coined the term "Type A" to describe the kind of behavior they came to believe placed both men and women at increased risk for heart disease. Their Type-A hallmarks were impatience and hostility.

Are You Type A?

Check your behavior against the following list. Type A's typically:

- Try to do two things at once—working while eating, reading while talking on the phone.
- Have a fixation about being on time.
- Have trouble sitting still and doing nothing.
- Yell at the stupidity of other drivers.
- Get irritated standing in lines.
- Interrupt people frequently.
- Always play to win, even in games with children.
- Have often been told by their spouses to slow down, and dismiss such exhortations as ridiculous or impossible.

In a now-classic series of experiments starting in 1960 and culminating in their 1974 best-seller, *Type A Behavior and Your Heart*, Dr. Friedman and Dr. Rosenman showed that compared with more relaxed Type B's, hostile, impatient, time-pressured Type A's were at substantially greater risk for heart attack. Ten years later, in *Treating Type-A Behavior and Your Heart*, Dr. Friedman and coauthor Diane Ulmer, R.N., showed that with intensive group therapy, Type A's who had suffered heart attacks could get off the hostility/impatience merry-go-round, dramatically reduce their risk of heart attack recurrence, and learn to lighten up, smell the roses, and enjoy life in ways they never before thought possible. The weekly counseling sessions include homework exercises designed to introduce stressed-out Type A's to the more laid-back side of life:

- Listen to your spouse. Stop arguing with requests to slow down.
- The next time you see someone doing a task more slowly than you could, do not interfere.
- Never interrupt anyone.
- Read a long novel far removed from your occupation.
- Purposely choose to wait in the longest line at the supermarket or toll plaza and use the time to reflect on what you enjoy about your life.

- Write a letter to an old friend. Do not mention your job. Use a thesaurus at least once.
- Laugh at yourself at least twice a day.

Firsthand Experience

For Dr. Meyer Friedman, treating Type-A behavior was much more than simply a way to win research grants. "You must understand," he says, "I have a classic Type-A personality. During World War II, my nickname was 'Cannonball Mike.' I never walked. I always ran. I was constantly in a rush, impatient and insecure. I'd get furious standing in lines. And you should have been me behind the wheel!" Dr. Friedman also has a long history of heart disease. In 1965 he suffered a heart attack, and in 1972 he had triple bypass surgery. Now 78, and as mellow a man as you're likely to meet, Dr. Friedman says he still has a Type-A personality.

"In my experience, you can't change your fundamental personality. But you *can* change your behavior." Like the Type A's who have been through his counseling program, Dr. Friedman has developed what he calls an "internal monitor," a little part of his consciousness that sees him as a stranger would see him, and constantly reminds him to relax, slow down, smile, forgive, and focus on what's really important without becoming wrought up over meaningless details. The "stranger" part is crucial. "If your monitor sees you as you're seen by your spouse or friends," he says, "you can always rationalize your anger and impatience. Strangers are much rougher judges of behavior. They don't know you, so they don't make excuses for you. They just see your behavior, and if it's hostile or impatient, they notice."

Years ago when Dr. Friedman first began transforming his Type-A behavior, one of his most difficult challenges was to break a lifelong habit of overscheduling his time. At first he had a hard time saying no to anything but eventually his monitor began asserting itself. "Every time a possible commitment presented itself—a meeting, concert, dinner, or speaking engagement—my monitor would ask if I'd care about the event after five years. If the answer were yes, I'd go. If not, I'd decline. When you take a five-year view, it really puts things in perspective. Try it. You'll be amazed at how trivial most social engagements are. Once I started turning down events that were ultimately meaningless to me, I found I had a lot more time for the things I considered really important, like friends and family, and my research."

Of course, Dr. Friedman's road to Type-B behavior has had its share of ruts, and his monitor is still far from perfect. He says he no longer has any trouble waiting in long lines, and never yells at other drivers anymore. But his old Type-A patterns reassert themselves when he sees unfairness—especially if he believes it's directed at him.

A couple of years ago, Dr. Friedman's monitor was sorely tested by the publication *The Trusting Heart: Great News about Type-A Behavior*, by Redford Williams, M.D., a behavioral medicine specialist at Duke. Dr. Williams's book essentially accuses Dr. Friedman of misleading the public about Type-A behavior. Dr. Williams claims impatience, ambition, and a time-pressured lifestyle have nothing to do with heart attack risk, that hostility is the only truly damaging Type-A personality trait. Dr. Williams's message is, go ahead, be a workaholic, be driven and time pressured. Just don't get angry about it.

When *The Trusting Heart* came out, Dr. Friedman's phone began ringing off the hook: *Time, Newsweek*, the *New York Times*, CBS News—everyone wanted him to respond to Dr. Williams's attacks on his original vision of Type-A behavior.

"At the time," Dr. Friedman recalls, "I hadn't met Dr. Williams, and I hadn't even seen his book. But his criticisms seemed terribly unfair to me. How can you separate impatience from hostility? When you feel impatient waiting in line, isn't that a form of hostility? And how could Dr. Williams say I criticized ambition? I never said ambition, per se, was necessarily Type A. I simply said Type A's *use* their ambitions in self-destructive ways. I must admit I got upset."

Fortunately, Dr. Friedman's monitor intervened and calmed him down. "Instead of getting angry and defensive, my monitor showed me another way to look at this problem. By targeting hostility, Dr. Williams was actually confirming our work. He was promoting our results. Thanks to my monitor, I was able to see that Williams and I mostly agreed with each other. We simply disagreed abut the relative importance of some of the details. I still think he's wrong about impatience, but that doesn't really matter. Since then, I've met Dr. Williams and read his book. And you know something? I like him. He's a good man."

I came away thinking Dr. Friedman's notion of a five-year perspective made a lot of sense. It helped me separate the wheat from the chaff in my own little stress drama. But Dr. Meyer Friedman could be my father. I wanted to speak with someone my own age, who had the same kinds of problems I had: job headaches, a growing family, a two-career marriage, and the horror of San Francisco Bay Area housing costs.

Healthy Pleasures

David Sobel, M.D., looks younger than his 41 years. In addition to maintaining a crowded medical practice, he is the Regional Director for Patient Education and Health Promotion of Northern California Kaiser-Permanente. He regularly covers a territory stretching hundreds of miles and spends a great deal of time on the road. For three years he was the medical correspondent on a San Jose television station and a frequent medical guest on "Hour Magazine," a nationally syndicated television program. Not to mention that he spends a good deal of time most days taking care of his three-year-old son, Matthew. Then there are Dr. Sobel's books. He and coauthor Robert Ornstein, Ph.D., have written *The Healing Brain* and *Healthy Pleasures*. Both books required months of painstaking research and deal in part with the mind/body connection, a subject that embraces the field of stress management.

As if Dr. Sobel's life weren't stressful enough, during one 18-month period, he had to contend with the unexpected death of a family member, and he and his wife had several rooms added to their San Jose home. In addition to enduring the millions of hassles typically involved in gutting one's home and rebuilding it from the inside out, the renovations were so extensive that Dr. Sobel and his family had to move out for two months, then move back in when the work was completed.

"It was quite a time," Dr. Sobel says with only a hint of weariness. "Very stressful. But that's life."

How does he cope? "Frankly," he says, "I don't worry much about managing my stress. I don't use any specific techniques. I'm not opposed to formal stress-management programs or exercises; some people need them. But I'm not involved in any. I simply try to fill my life with activities I personally find pleasurable, things that help rejuvenate me.

"There's nothing I find more restorative than playing with my son. I was raised to view time spent doing child care as 'nonproductive.' But that's simply not true. Playing with Matthew is probably the most stress-managing thing in my life. Of course, he can also be a pain. But research we cite in *The Healing Brain* and *Healthy Pleasures* is quite clear. People who are deeply involved in themselves and their careers need some focus outside themselves: children, hobbies, gardening—whatever. And conversely, people who give a great deal of their energy to others, for example full-time mothers, need to balance those commitments with time they reserve just for themselves."

Part of the personal balancing act Dr. Sobel practices involves what psychologists call developing "self-complexity," a multifaceted personality. "Self-complexity is another way of saying that variety is the spice of life," Dr. Sobel explains. "The more complex you are, the more friends, hobbies, and diverse interests you have, the better defended you are against the stresses of adversity. Most people like to see themselves as one unified person, and the media make a big deal out of people who devote themselves entirely to some 'magnificent obsession.' But people who become obsessed with anything generally lose perspective on everything else, and fundamentally, stress management is the ability to place your problems in the context of the larger world. I'm not saying you shouldn't be committed to your work. It's great to love your work and give 100 percent. But nobody's work goes well all the time. And when things in one part of your life go badly, it really helps to have some good things happening in other parts. Maybe you had a fight with your boss, but if your flowers are blooming and your softball team is on a winning streak, those outside interests can help keep the job problems in perspective."

Dr. Sobel says a great deal of stress management boils down to time-honored adages like "count your blessings," which stress-management authorities call "the stories we tell ourselves." "Stress, per se, is not the problem," he insists. "It's how we react to our stressors that causes our problems. In the last year and a half, I've been hit with a terrible family tragedy. I've remodeled my house, which involved lots of stress. And I've had a book deadline and other headaches as well. If I sit down and tell myself that my life is an endless litany of problems and tragedies, all I can do is get depressed—significantly increase my risk for stress-related illness. But if I tell myself that my wife and I are healthy, that we have a good marriage and a wonderful son, that we're building the home we always dreamed of and, oh yes, that we also have the same kinds of problems and tragedies everyone else has to deal with, then I don't get depressed. I can keep things in perspective. I certainly wouldn't wish personal tragedy on anyone, but the death in my family really put things in perspective for me. The worst problems with our remodeling job became trivial by comparison."

But David Sobel is a doctor, a professional in a high-status job. What about assembly-line workers and burger flippers at McDonald's? How can they deal with their stress? "Job stress isn't just related to the type of work you do," Dr. Sobel says. "It depends a lot on how much control you have over your work. My job is very demanding, but I have a reasonable amount of control over it, so as jobs go, it's not all that stressful—even though it feels very stressful at times. The same is true for most corporate management jobs. When you say 'stress,' people usually think of executives, but their jobs are not really that stressful. The most stressful jobs make big demands but allow little control, for example, assembly-line work. Factories are more productive when the workers get more control, so I think the trend toward worker/management teamwork is helpful. But it's not enough. Jobs that limit people's control also erode their self-esteem. Nobody likes to feel like a drone. That's why it's doubly important for people in high-stress jobs to develop outside interests they love, interests that nurture their self-esteem.

"One thing that really helps is volunteer work helping those less fortunate than yourself. Volunteer work is an old-time folksy approach to stress management. Put another way, there are a lot of selfish reasons to be altruistic. In addition to the good that comes from the volunteering itself, assisting people in dire straits helps the helpers keep their own problems in perspective. It also boosts their self-esteem."

Dr. Sobel's book, *Healthy Pleasures,* emerged in part from his observation that social scientists have spent too much time studying people who are unhappy. "Happiness," he says, "is just another way of saying you have your stress load under control. So asking what makes people happy is a good way to learn what helps them manage their stress. When you ask what would make them happy, most people's initial response is 'more money.' Now if you're poor, or homeless, and can't feed or clothe your family, extra money makes a tremendous contribution to happiness. But if your basic life needs are met, more money doesn't really add all that much to happiness. Every survey of lottery winners has shown the same thing: One year after they've hit the jackpot, after the initial euphoria has worn off, they're not particularly happier than they were before they struck it rich. Maybe they bought a Mercedes. But as time passes, they're not much happier with the Mercedes than they were with the old Ford.

"Beyond health, family, and friends, and having your basic needs met, it's not the big things in life that make the difference. It's the little pleasures you create for yourself: playing with your kids, phone calls to old friends, a hug, a compliment, gardening, having pets, gazing into an aquarium. We have a chocolate-colored Burmese cat, Coco. Having her purr on my lap feels more relaxing to me than most formal stress-management programs. We also recently purchased an aquarium. I absolutely love it. We have angel fish, fantail guppies, and a bala shark.

Staring into an aquarium puts you in touch with a whole different realm of existence. It's amazingly relaxing."

Dr. Sobel also keeps things in perspective with the help of a globe and world maps displayed around his home. "Whenever I get upset about something in my little corner of the world, I spin my globe. San Jose is a tiny dot. California is a little sliver. It's a big world out there, and each of us is just a microscopic part of it."

An aquarium. Hmmm. My wife and I have been scuba divers for years and love to watch fish. Maybe something like that would help me find a measure of peace. . . . But Dr. Sobel works for a huge institution. Lord knows that's not easy, but he's not really in touch with the kinds of small-business challenges I face. So I visited Esther Orioli, an entrepreneur who runs a small business.

Toy Dinosaurs

"The bad news," Orioli says with a wry smile, "is that reality is the cause of all stress. The good news is that most of us aren't in touch with it."

The 38-year-old, curly-haired founder and president of Essi Systems, Inc., of San Francisco, is something of a maverick in the world of stress management. She dislikes being called a "stress expert." Her Master's degree is an offbeat field, adult education. And she doesn't see stress as necessarily negative. In fact, she often celebrates its positive benefits, a view that has landed her in hot water with some of the field's Big Guns.

Over the last two decades, Esther Orioli has taught high-school English, run a community-college career development office, and been the director of several alcohol- and drug-abuse treatment and prevention programs. She stumbled into stress management by accident in 1981 during a stint as a partner in a firm that coordinated Employee Assistance Programs for several large San Francisco Area corporations. Her partners were committed to their alcohol- and drug-abuse work, but Orioli got seriously bitten by the stress-management bug and decided to found her own company to pursue her new passion. The "Essi" in Essi Systems, Inc. was her childhood nickname.

"I was trained as a teacher," Orioli says, "and I've always taught what I most needed to learn." She launched Essi Systems in 1983 on a wing and a prayer and set out "to do something with stress." But she didn't know what. Through her work in Employee Assistance, she'd met two Bay Area psychologists, Dennis Jaffe, Ph.D, and Cynthia Scott, Ph.D., who'd been toying with the idea of developing a new-and-improved personal stress inventory. "All the 'Rate Your Stress' quizzes you see in the popular magazines are too simplistic," Orioli said. "They treat stress like some kind of disease. If you have 'stress,' it's like you have 'germs.' You're sick, and the only way to get well is to get rid of all your stress. But that's not the way it works. Sure, some stress produces negative reactions: anxiety, tension, burnout, illness. But stress is a normal part of life. Its effects occur along a continuum. There are certainly negatives at one end, but there's a positive side to stress as well: passion, excitement, determination, thrills. Without stress, we wouldn't have surprise parties, murder mysteries, and roller coasters. Life wouldn't be worth living."

Orioli teamed up with Dr. Jaffe and Dr. Scott to develop a personal stress inventory that would tell both sides of the stress story, one that would alert people to the parts of their lives causing strain and burnout, but also pinpoint the areas where their coping skills had allowed them to achieve balance and optimal performance.

In 1984, the trio completed the prototype for their stress test, and Orioli borrowed $90,000 from friends and relatives to self-publish it under the name StressMap. That was when the stress level at Essi Systems went from balance to near-burnout. Orioli set to work building her company around marketing her new product, but when the boxes were delivered, Orioli stood staring at floor-to-ceiling stacks of StressMaps, all unsold, knowing she had big bucks in loans to repay.

Fortunately for Orioli, over the last several years, her view that stress can be a motivator as well as a nemesis has helped her—and the half-dozen people who now work for Essi Systems—sell more than 100,000 StressMaps to such heavy hitters as AT&T, Apple Computer, Levi Strauss, Clorox, Lockheed, and Sharper Image. Orioli re-

paid the $90,000 on schedule, but as anyone in the entre-
preneurial world knows, running your own company is
no picnic. She has faced organizational growing pains,
legal problems, financial challenges, and a move to larger
offices—with another expansion in the offing.

Although Essi Systems has been consistently profitable,
Orioli has been unable to get bank financing, partly, she
is convinced, because she is a woman. So she turned to
venture capitalists, who were very interested, "but they
wanted 70 percent of Essi stock, and told me they'd have
to replace me with a man. I said, 'No way,' and developed
my own alternative financing plan, something I call cre-
ative financing. It involves private loans from one's personal network." Orioli is now in the process of developing
a Play Bank Kit to sell to other entrepreneurs.

"I love my life," Orioli says, "and I've consciously created
it to allow me to head my own company and do the work I
like to do. But I have negative stress, too. Who doesn't? I
carry my 'distress' in knots in my neck and shoulders, in
shallow breathing, and in rapid-fire talking. I try to pay attention to those signs, and when I feel any of them happening, I take immediate action. A sore neck is my body's way
of whispering to me that I have some work to do. The body
whispers before it shouts. I try to listen and cope with negative stress before burnout sets in."

For her neck and shoulders, Orioli gets a weekly mas-
sage and goes for long walks with friends. Whenever she
feels herself slipping into shallow breathing, she sings or
plays the harmonica. "The world of stress management is
filled with breathing exercises, but frankly, I need something more personal, something that works for me. Singing and playing harmonica are fun and they accomplish
the same thing as any deep-breathing exercises. I even
keep a harmonica in my car and pull it out when I'm stuck
in traffic."

Orioli concedes she's "bad about exercise. That's supposed to be embarrassing for a 'stress' expert to admit, but
I find it impossible to go home, change into a jogging
outfit, then go out again and run. Whatever it takes to be
a runner, I don't have it." As an alternative, she's developed a more personal form of exercise which she uses as

an after-work transition ritual. "I love jazz and I love to dance. Recently, I bought a CD player and pulled most of the furniture out of my living room to give me a big open studio space. When I come home, I put on some Grover Washington or Sarah Vaughn or Gato Barbieri and dance. It really helps me feel balanced and centered."

She's also weaned herself from a lifelong obsession with the news. "I used to read three newspapers a day and watch the 11 o'clock news every night. But most news is bad news. It's made up of events I'm powerless to change. Feeling powerless is a real negative stressor for me, so I've stopped being so news focused. I believe in being reasonably well informed, so I still read one newspaper a day, but that's all."

Finally, Orioli has her prized toy dinosaur collection. "I don't know why, but I've always loved little toy dinosaurs. Some people have pets; I have my dinosaurs. I keep some at work. I have more at home. And when I travel, I take a few along. Call me crazy, but I just feel safer and happier with them around."

The final element in Orioli's own stress-management program is what one might call her mantra. When things get tough, she repeats it to herself over and over again: Don't sweat the small stuff. And it's all small stuff.

Happy Ending

Recently, my stress situation has smoothed out considerably. I've taken some of Dr. Meyer Friedman's advice. I try to see everyday demands in a five-year perspective. When overscheduling puts me into a nasty funk, I go with the commitment I'll care about in five years. That's given me more time for friends, family, and gardening.

Meanwhile, I've followed Dr. David Sobel's lead and taken the plunge into aquarium ownership. It took a while to get our tank functioning. At first my wife and I killed an appalling number of fish. Then we got our pH karma together, and now we have a respectable aquarium, including a red-tail shark, which is all of an inch long, but it reminds me of the white-tip reef sharks we saw while diving in Fiji. One glance at the tank, and I'm back at 60 feet gliding over the cabbage coral in the Somo Somo Strait.

Finally, inspired by Esther Orioli, I've been expanding my CD collection. After a tough day of editing, I drop into the local record store and peruse the compact disks. If you're into new rock, "The Raw and the Cooked" by the Fine Young Cannibals is terrific. I'd also recommend anything by Ry Cooder.

As fate would have it, Bobby McFerrin lives in my San Francisco neighborhood, and I spotted him in the record store one day shortly after he'd won the Grammy for "Don't Worry, Be Happy." People congratulated him, and he smiled back, a friendly, ingratiating smile, but on closer inspection, not an entirely happy one—more like the way you smile at 2 A.M. on your wedding night as the band is packing up and you're standing around the suddenly empty hall kissing the last of your bride's third cousins good night—a smile that silently spoke volumes about frayed nerves and strained coping abilities.

I considered offering my services as a newly enlightened stress expert, but I figured McFerrin would prefer to be left alone. Instead I picked up a copy of "Don't Worry, Be Happy." Bobby has a great voice, and on CD it really sparkles.

CHAPTER 23

Vision Quests

Advances in the prevention and treatment of middle- to older-age problems can keep your sight right on target.

Looking into the future of vision care for aging eyes, the prospects are encouraging: Chances are better than ever that you will be able to enjoy good vision well into your golden years.

It's true that your eyes age along with the rest of you,

and vision-stealing problems become more troublesome beginning in the middle years. But thanks to bold new advances in research, ophthalmologists now wield an array of innovative techniques and powerfully precise instruments that can help preserve our precious sight.

Good News about Glaucoma

The most common threat to good vision in midlife is glaucoma—the buildup of damaging fluid pressure inside your eyeballs. Two out of every 100 people over age 35 suffer from glaucoma. Your chances of getting it zoom if someone else in your family has glaucoma, if you are black, or if you have diabetes, hardening of the arteries, or anemia.

Here's what happens: No one knows exactly why, but your eyes' drainage system can start to clog over the years, so the fluid in your eyeball, called the aqueous humor, backs up. The fluid's pressure can ravage the delicate nerves inside your eyes, probably by cutting off their blood supply. Glaucoma steals side vision first and can eventually blind you.

Bringing eye pressure down to safe levels and keeping it down can halt glaucoma damage but nothing can restore already wrecked nerves. Fortunately, breakthroughs have improved both fluid-pressure control and glaucoma diagnosis.

The Molteno implant. Once this device is implanted in your eye, it acts like a tiny plastic faucet. Fluid automatically flows out whenever pressure starts to build up inside your eye. The Molteno implant offers new hope to glaucoma victims whose eye pressure resists control by drugs or surgery.

The implant consists of a ½-inch circular acrylic anchoring plate attached to a ¾-inch-long silicone drainage tube that can be placed in your eye during a 40-minute, one-day hospital procedure, according to Jeffrey Freedman, M.D., professor of clinical ophthalmology at the State University of New York Health Science Center at Brooklyn. Several years ago Dr. Freedman was the only surgeon in America using Molteno implants, but nowadays the procedure is performed by 50 to 60 ophthalmologists across the country.

The surgeon injects a local anesthetic into the conjunctiva, the colorless skin that covers the white of the eye. Looking through a surgical microscope, he cuts open and folds back a flap of conjunctiva. He then sews the implant's plate onto your eye's white, or sclera, to anchor the drainage tube. He inserts one end of the tube into your eyeball and positions the other end behind your eye so your body can absorb any fluid that drains out. To tuck the tube into place, the surgeon stitches a covering of scleral tissue taken from a donor eye. Finally, he sews the conjunctiva closed.

The Molteno implant is not obvious in your eye unless you lift your upper lid, exposing the raised area over the tube. The stitches are so fine you can't feel them, and they stay in permanently. You apply a combination antibiotic and steroid drop to your eye for six weeks after the procedure, but an eye patch is unnecessary. Redness disappears after ten days to two weeks, and in a week or two your vision returns to normal.

Ocusert eye-drop dispenser. Ocusert is a prescription-drug dispenser made by Alza Corporation. It's a tiny contact-lens-like wafer that sits on the sclera under the lower eyelid so it doesn't block vision. The dispenser steadily discharges the prescribed medication, making eye-pressure control easier and more exact for some glaucoma victims.

You insert a new Ocusert wafer each week, using a technique much like inserting a contact lens: After washing and drying your hands, you hold the wafer on your index finger, pull your lower lid down and lay the wafer on the white of your eye.

Some of the drawbacks: Ocusert costs more than eye drops, its presence in your eye may be difficult to adjust to, and it may drop out of your eye, especially during sleep.

Ocusert is an option only if your doctor prescribes pilocarpine, one of several glaucoma drugs. It works best for less severe types of glaucoma, according to Thomas Hutchinson, M.D., glaucoma specialist at Harvard Medical School.

This new medication delivery system is especially useful because people with glaucoma are supposed to use eye drops up to four times a day every day to keep fluid pressure steady and ward off nerve damage. But in a recent study of 184 glaucoma patients, one-quarter missed an entire day of medication each month and 30 percent used an entire day's dosage in a short period instead of throughout the day, as directed.

New early-diagnosis exam. Until recently, doctors scouting for signs of glaucoma were limited to looking for telltale pitting on the main optic nerve where it enters the back of your eyeball. But then researchers discovered that you can have seemingly normal eye pressure, no vision problems and a healthy-looking optic nerve yet still have signs of damage in the layer of nerve fibers that branch out from the main nerve. This new technique uncovers glaucoma clues in the fine web of nerve fibers lining the inside of your eyeball. Most ophthalmologists now do this exam in their office.

George Baerveldt, M.D., associate professor of ophthalmology at the Doheny Eye Institute in Los Angeles, describes the procedure: First, your doctor uses various instruments to help him see inside your eye. Then he shines a special green light into your eye to illuminate the nerve fibers. Your doctor can spot tiny slits where fluid pressure has destroyed the fibers. He photographs the inside of your eye as a basis for comparing results with any future exams. The whole procedure takes about 10 minutes and is painless, although the camera flashes can be annoying.

New Tricks for Old Eyes

Somewhere around age 45, when you find yourself squinting at newsprint held at arm's length, you'll have achieved a middle-age milestone: presbyopia, the lessening of ability to focus at near distances. The problem is probably due to loss of the lenses' flexibility or a weakening of the tiny muscles suspending them. This condition differs from farsightedness, which is not age related. In farsighted people, the eye is somewhat shorter than it needs to be, so light rays focus beyond the retina.

No one escapes presbyopia. The decline actually starts in your first decade of life. "Fine work you could do 3 inches away at 8 years old, you'd have to do at 3½ inches at 15, and at 5 inches at age 20," says George Weinstein,

M.D., ophthalmology department chairman at West Virginia University.

Bifocal contact lenses. Diffractive bifocal contact lenses provide an innovative solution to those who need help seeing both near and far and would rather wear contacts than bifocal eyeglasses. Most candidates are nearsighted and are already wearing contacts or glasses to see far away when presbyopia starts to smudge their near vision.

Diffractive lenses work like this: At the center of each contact is a bull's-eye of circular lenses. Each ring is less than one-twentieth the diameter of a human hair and each splits the light entering your eye in two. The result is that your eye receives two images at all times—one near and one far—and your brain decides which one to recognize for close-up or distant vision.

That may sound like a recipe for a headache, but experts say your brain can handle the strain. The lenses do have two weaknesses: Because you have only half the available light for closeup vision, you may find reading difficult in a dim room. Also, some wearers see faint halos around lights, which makes nighttime driving difficult.

Diffractive bifocal lenses are soft and use standard soft-contact-lens cleaning systems. Allergan Optical Company manufactures the only diffractive bifocal lenses available in this country, under the brand name Echelon.

Researchers have been tinkering with bifocal contacts for years, but the earlier designs just didn't work, says Oliver H. Dabezies, M.D., a contact-lens specialist at Tulane University Medical Center, in New Orleans. Another cosmetic alternative to bifocals is the new generation of glasses made without the age-betraying dividing line separating the top and bottom halves of the lens. Your eye doctor can tell you how to get a pair.

Ready-to-wear eyeglasses. Good news for your eyes and your pocketbook: Those inexpensive reading glasses for sale in drugstores and five-and-dimes have been declared "medically acceptable, cost-effective, and in the best overall interest of the public" by the American Academy of Ophthalmology (AAO).

The AAO has determined that you can't hurt your eyes by trying ready-to-wears on your own. If your vision is otherwise good when presbyopia strikes, all you need are glasses that magnify print or fine work. If you have another, undetected vision problem that requires prescription glasses, you'll discover it when the over-the-counter reading glasses don't help you. And reading glasses must meet federal safety requirements to resist breaking if you are struck in the face, just as prescription glasses must. "Even some ophthalmologists have started stocking inexpensive reading glasses for their presbyopic patients," says Dr. Weinstein, secretary of the AAO's public and professional information committee. But while you're saving a few dollars by avoiding prescription glasses for presbyopia, warns Dr. Weinstein, don't shortchange yourself on regular eye exams that can catch other middle-age eye disorders. (The AAO recommends you have a medical eye exam at age 40, then every two to five years later.)

Cataract Breakthroughs

Like presbyopia, cataracts are a common occurrence with advancing age. The prevailing theory is that over a period of years ultraviolet sunlight triggers chemical reactions within the lens of the eye, blocking out the light. Recent studies suggest that the more ultraviolet rays your eyes are exposed to over your lifetime, the sooner cataracts may cloud your eyes. That's why the AAO recommends you wear brimmed hats and sunglasses whenever you're outdoors.

The remedy for cataracts is to remove the offending lenses, and over one million cataract surgeries are done in the United States each year. For the last eight or nine years, cataract treatment for 90 percent of patients consisted of surgery to insert an artificial replacement lens.

Preventive laser scans. Now there's exciting potential for heading off cataracts in the making. A new low-level laser device still in experimental stages can spot the first traces of cataract-forming proteins in your lenses and measure how fast they're growing. Combined with an experimental drug that may stop or reverse protein production, this technology holds out the first promise of delaying cataracts—and the surgery to remove them—for as long as 15 to 20 years.

Laser scanning uses a small tabletop device with a cord containing two fiber-optic wires—narrow plastic tubes that transmit laser beams. You just sit in your doctor's chair while he scans each lens using a penlike device at the end of the cord. Laser beams fired from one fiberoptic thread bounce off any protein molecules present and are collected by the other tube leading back to the device. There the results are analyzed and fed to your doctor. A 5-second scan in each eye is all it takes.

Cataract-predicting lasers are nothing like the burning lasers used in some types of eye surgery. According to developer Nai-Teng Yu, M.D., at Georgia Institute of Technology, this laser is only one-thirtieth as intense as the light from a standard ophthalmoscope.

Dr. Yu, who's an adjunct ophthalmology professor at Emory University, in Atlanta, has tested the laser scanner on donated human lenses in his lab. He's now using the device in a two-year study to track the effectiveness of an experimental cataract-slowing drug in diabetics at the Joslin Diabetes Center in Boston. Dr. Yu says doctors could be using his laser to screen high-risk patients—like diabetics—within the next few years.

Higher-tech surgery. Many doctors are taking advantage of technological advances to streamline cataract surgery from start to finish, according to the AAO's Dr. Weinstein.

Pressure-lowering devices used before surgery help reduce pressure in your eye so a surgeon can operate without causing damage to eye tissue. After a numbing injection, your doctor places a band around your head that positions a rubber ball over the eye to be operated on. Your eye responds by releasing some of its fluid within a few minutes, dropping the pressure inside.

Viscoelastic gels hold delicate tissues away from the scalpel, adding an extra margin of safety to operations within your eyeball's close quarters. Your surgeon may insert some of this gooey material after his opening incision to protect your iris, the colored part of your eye, for example. Viscoelastic gels are inactive and can remain in your eye after the surgery.

Relief
from Diabetic Blindness

If you have diabetes, your vision faces a unique threat: retinopathy—the weakening and leaking of the blood vessels lining the retina. Midlife can be treacherous because your risk of retinopathy increases with time. Sixty percent of people who've had diabetes for 15 years have damage to the blood vessels of the eye.

Normal blood flow nourishes the retina, the portion of your eye where light focuses. Blood, proteins, and fats that may escape the vessels can cause swelling and damage your retina, so the picture sent to your brain becomes blurred. In some cases, retinopathy robs you of the ability to read and drive. But in one victim out of five, retinopathy progresses to the second, proliferative stage in which there's bleeding into the center of your eye. This can cause loss of vision if treatment isn't started in time.

Standard treatment for retinopathy involves using a laser to create scars in the retina, which reduces the chance of bleeding, according to Ronald Klein, M.D., ophthalmology professor at the University of Wisconsin Medical School.

"Roto-Rooter" rescue. In an operation called vitrectomy, your doctor places Lilliputian instruments inside your eye, using a high-power surgical microscope to view the back of the eye. He can then remove the blood that's hemorrhaged into your eye's interior and repair retinal tears if necessary.

Vitrectomy is done by a surgeon in the hospital under general or local anesthesia. Pillows are positioned to hold your head motionless, and the surgeon rests his hands on your face to steady them. Peering through the microscope, the surgeon makes three tiny incisions into your eyes in a narrow zone just outside the colored part, then he threads his instruments through the holes.

Into one hole goes a fiberoptic instrument to light up the inside of your eye and to look around. Into the second goes a tube to infuse a saltwater mixture (identical to your body's fluid) to keep your eye from collapsing. The third is the "working" hole through which the surgeon inserts miniature instruments.

The surgeon then removes the blood or blood-soaked tissue by using the vitrectomy suction-cutter, described as a minuscule "Roto-Rooter," by Andrew J. Packer, M.D., an ophthalmologic surgeon at the Hartford Hospital Eye Institute, in Connecticut. Through the working hole, the surgeon may also insert a laser probe to treat the unhealthy blood vessels that proliferate in the second phase of retinopathy. Or the surgeon may do other repair work with tiny forceps or scissors.

The vitrectomy takes 2 to 3 hours and ends with the surgeon closing the three holes with stitches that dissolve as your eye heals. Your doctor will give you antibiotic ointment to smear on your eye for several weeks and drops to keep your pupil in the dilated and rested position. A patch is often unnecessary, but Dr. Packer recommends his patients wear sunglasses to reduce the light entering their dilated eyes, for comfort's sake. Vitrectomy is now performed in hospitals throughout the country.

Repairing Detached Retinas

The vitreous humor, the gel that fills up the inside of your eyeball, sticks to the retina. As your eyes age, the vitreous humor may pucker and pull away from the inside surface of your eye, detaching the retina from your eye wall. The detached retina leaves a blind spot in the picture your retina transmits to your brain.

Retinal detachment happens to 1 in 10,000 people every year, usually in middle age or later. To repair the damage, your doctor may have to do a vitrectomy or scleral buckle (attaching an elastic band to the outside of the eye to force the eye wall back against the retina). But if the detachment is uncomplicated, he may decide to try an ingenious repair technique that restores vision in 30 minutes.

Less-invasive air repair. Pneumatic retinopexy involves injecting air into your eye to gently press your retina back against the eye wall. Unlike vitrectomy, few incisions are made into your eyeball.

After administering an injection to numb your eye, the doctor looks inside your eye with an ophthalmoscope. He locates and treats the tear with either a laser or a freezing application.

He then injects a bubble of air into your vitreous humor. The whole procedure takes half an hour or even less. The air bubble lasts for about a week until your normal eyeball fluid replaces it.

Here's the only drawback to air injection: Because the technique depends on pressure from the air bubble, you must spend most of the next five to seven days with your head in a fixed position. Depending on the site of the tear, you may have to sit with your head resting on a table or lie facedown in bed to keep the bubble positioned over the tear.

The up side is, you can be back to work in a week or two, compared to a six-week layoff following a vitrectomy, according to Michael Gaynon, M.D., researcher at the Stanford University Hospital. In a study of 198 people treated for detached retinas, those who had air injection recovered faster and enjoyed better vision than those who had the traditional procedure. Air injection is being done by retinal surgeons in many hospitals and private offices.

Hope
for Macular Degeneration

For over three million Americans, reading, sewing, even recognizing familiar faces is a challenge because the center of their vision is permanently blurred. That's because of a breakdown in the macula—the portion of the eye that light falls on when looking straight ahead. Beginning at about age 50, blood vessels behind the macula may start to leak fluid, creating sight-obscuring scar tissue.

There is no cure for macular degeneration, although lasers can corral one form of it, keeping it from spreading out into your retina by sealing off leaky blood vessels. While scientists continue their search for ways to battle this disorder, one group of researchers has uncovered a potentially powerful predictor of who will develop macular degeneration years before it starts.

Red-light signals. In the near future, a new visual function test may be able to measure your response to a flashing red light to gauge your risk for macular degeneration. It enlists equipment that's already standard in your eye doctor's office.

First, your doctor gives you pupil-dilating eye drops in the test eye, then he puts a patch over it for 45 minutes to make your eye supersensitive to the test light.

The room is then darkened, and the patch comes off. Your doctor gives you a target of four dots in a diamond shape to stare at to focus his aim at your macula. In the center of the diamond, a red light flashes off and on. Each flash is slightly dimmer than the last. For each flash you see you press a buzzer. The last—and faintest—red flash you report measures your macula's sensitivity. Your doctor uses that information to calculate your risk for macular degeneration.

In a pilot study of 18 people 55 years and older, the red light test accurately identified the five people who developed macular degeneration during the following four years. Janet S. Sunness, M.D., researcher at the Wilmer Institute, Johns Hopkins University Medical School, has begun a larger study of the test.

CHAPTER 24

Is Your Medication Zapping Your Hair?

Most doctors don't even know that many common drugs cause hair loss. Here's a guide to help you identify the culprits.

There's a hairy little secret no one in the pharmaceutical industry wants to discuss. A surprising number of popular medications can cause hair loss, but all the drug companies want to talk about is hair growth.

Hair growth is hot. One recent drug ad shows a man staring pensively across a beach. At the back of his head, a developing bald spot is clearly visible. The headline says, "If you're concerned about hair loss . . . see your doctor." Although no product is named, it's an ad for Upjohn's Rogaine Topical Solution (minoxidil), the first baldness remedy to win Food and Drug Administration (FDA) approval.

Clearly, hair loss is an emotional issue. Until recently, dermatologists believed nothing could be done for male pattern baldness (alopecia). Now that's all changed. Minoxidil doesn't work for everyone, but it works well enough for the FDA, and now many drug companies are researching hair growth stimulants.

However, few drug industry spokespeople ever mention that many prescription drugs may cause hair to thin, and doctors rarely mention baldness as a potential side effect. Many physicians don't realize it's possible.

When patients discover through their own experience that their medicine makes their hair fall out, the emotional consequences can be devastating. Here's what one woman said in a letter to *Prevention:* "I hope you can point me to a blood pressure drug that doesn't cause hair loss. I am partially bald as an adverse reaction to blood pressure medicines, and I find some cholesterol-lowering drugs do the same thing.

"These medications may lower my blood pressure and cholesterol, but they are ruining my self-esteem. When I look in the mirror, my blood pressure soars. Isn't there any drug that won't affect my hair?"

Baldness is a well-known consequence of many cancer chemotherapy medications. When treating potentially life-threatening diseases, most people are willing to put up with temporary hair loss. But in less dire circumstances— for example hypertension or elevated cholesterol—most people would prefer to be forewarned that their drugs might thin their hair.

A Partial List

Here are just a few of the commonly prescribed medications known to increase the risk of temporary baldness (reversible alopecia).

- The cholesterol-lowering drugs, clofibrate (Atromid-S) and gemfibrozil (Lopid)
- Many arthritis medications, including auranofin (Ridaura), indomethacin (Indocin), naproxen (Naprosyn), sulindac (Clinoril), and methotrexate (Folex)
- Beta-blocker blood pressure drugs such as atenolol (Tenormin), metroprolol (Lopressor), nadolol (Corgard), propranolol (Inderal), and timolol (Blocadren)
- And occasionally such commonly prescribed ulcer drugs as cimetidine (Tagamet), ranitidine (Zantac), and famotidine (Pepcid)

Other medications occasionally reported to be associated with hair loss include oral contraceptives, blood thinners, seizure medications, male hormones (anabolic steroids), and vitamin-A derived drugs including isotretinoin (Accutane) and etretinate (Tegison).

Ask the Right Questions

Drug industry spokespeople may not mention baldness as a side effect of common medications, but don't overlook this upsetting possibility. Next time your doctor prescribes any drug for you, ask if it's linked to hair loss. Your doctor may not know. Encourage him or her to look it up in the *Physicians' Desk Reference (PDR)*, which lists the side effects of all prescription medications. If the drug is linked to reversible alopecia, ask if another can be substituted. And just to make sure your physician has given you accurate information, when you get the prescription filled, ask your pharmacist as well.

CHAPTER 25

Fighting Athlete's Foot

By Anne Simons, M.D.

Home remedies can cure most cases of this most common fungal infection of the skin.

It itches and burns. It causes scaling and cracking between the toes and thickening of the skin elsewhere on the foot. People whose socks become sweaty because of poorly ventilated athletic shoes, and those who use school or health club locker room showers are particularly susceptible, hence the name. But "athlete's foot" is actually a misnomer on two counts. It is by no means limited to athletes. And the fungal family that causes it may infect many other areas of the skin.

Athlete's foot is a form of ringworm, which is not a worm, but a species of *Trichophyton* fungus. Doctors call *Trichophyton* infections "tinea." On the scalp, tinea causes hair loss and scaly patches. On the body, tinea appears as round, red, scaly, itchy patches. On the fingers, it often appears as itchy scales, or raised itchy bumps. In the groin area, tinea is usually called "jock itch," though women can get it, too. Between the legs, the infection causes itching and skin thickening. Athlete's foot is technically known as "tinea pedis." The particular *Trichophyton* species that usually cause it (*T. mentagrophytes* and *T. rubrum*) require a warm, moist environment—exactly what develops inside well-worn workout footwear.

Athlete's foot is by far the most common fungal infection of the skin. Approximately 4 percent of the population is infected at any given moment. Athlete's foot is almost seven times more prevalent among men—68 per 1,000 compared with 11 per 1,000 among women. The infection is more common in hot, humid weather. Some controversy surrounds its transmission, but most authorities believe the infection spreads by direct contact with contaminated locker room and bathroom floors. As a result, athlete's foot spreads easily among family, team, and health club members.

The most common symptom is itching (pruritus). Some people suffer only mild discomfort. Others may be driven to distraction. In severe cases, fissures open up between the toes, and fluid "weeps" from the openings. The skin becomes soft (macerated), and painful burning and stinging may accompany the basic itching. In severe cases, a secondary bacterial infection may complicate the athlete's foot infection, causing additional discomfort and unpleasant odor.

Prevention

Athlete's foot can often be treated without drugs, simply with some hygienic and lifestyle measures. Before you rush off to the drug store or doctor, invest a week or so in keeping your feet—especially the skin between your toes—as dry as possible. Air your feet often. Use thick, absorbent socks that wick perspiration away from the skin. Change socks often. Wear well-ventilated athletic shoes. If possible, wear sandals or open-toed shoes. Dust your feet and shoes with cornstarch, which helps absorb excess moisture. And wear thongs in bathrooms, locker rooms, and showers to avoid reinfection and spreading your athlete's foot to anyone else.

Treatment

If symptoms persist, try an over-the-counter (OTC) antifungal cream or powder. Most drug stores carry quite a few. Creams are more effective than powders, but powders help absorb moisture. FDA-approved active ingredients include miconazole nitrate (Micatin), tolnaftate (Aftate, Tinactin, Dr. Scholl's Athlete's Foot Cream), and undecylenic acid and/or zinc undecylenate (Desenex, Rid-Itch).

After washing and drying the feet completely, apply a thin layer once or twice a day between the toes and all over the feet. Product directions vary—follow package directions—but most recommended daily use for four weeks. Symptoms should begin to resolve within a few days, but continue using the product for the recommended duration to avoid recurrence.

Which active ingredient is best? All are effective. Experiment for yourself. Some people respond better to one than another. You might also try rotating OTC products. Some people respond best to a combination of ingredients.

If you shop at a chain drugstore, you may be able to save money by buying a house brand antifungal cream. At one neighborhood Thrifty, Jr. store, a half-ounce tube of a brand name product sells for $4.95, but Thrifty Antifungal Cream—with the identical concentration of the same active ingredient—sells for just $1.79.

If symptoms persist or recur after using an OTC product for about a month, your physician may prescribe a more potent topical antifungal cream such as ketoconazole (Nizoral) or clotrimazole (Lotrimin).

Finally, in persistent cases, take a look at your toenails. If they appear thickened and discolored (typically white), your athlete's foot may be complicated by a fungal toenail infection. Toenail infections do not respond to nondrug or OTC treatments. They require prescription medication, typically oral griseofulvin (Fulvicin, Grisactin). Treatment takes several months because the infected nail must grow out completely and be replaced by new healthy nail. Severe cases sometimes require surgical nail removal. If itching and any other athlete's foot symptoms persist during treatment, continue to use OTC products.

CHAPTER 26

Cure Chronic Hyperventilation

Experts estimate that as many as one in ten people visiting the doctor's office suffer from this breathing problem.

A crushing pain gripped George's chest. His heart raced. Sweat poured from his palms. He gulped for air. By all appearances, George was having a heart attack, the result of cholesterol-clogged arteries choking off the blood supply to his heart. But after a battery of tests, doctors ruled out heart disease. Apparently, George's "angina" pain and other symptoms were brought on by nothing more than hyperventilation.

Fast, Shallow Breathing

Hyperventilation is fast, shallow breathing. All of us do it at one time or another; it's considered a normal physiological response to stress—part of the so-called fight-or-flight response that saved our ancestors from saber-toothed tigers and the like. Usually, our breathing patterns return to normal once the threat passes.

But sometimes hyperventilation can become habitual. And, in most of these cases, neither the patient nor his doctor recognizes the problem. Because the symptoms associated with hyperventilation are broad and variable— including shortness of breath; light-headedness; tingling and coldness in the fingers, face, and feet; excessive sighing or yawning; belching; anxiety; fatigue; gastrointestinal symptoms; even chest pains—regular hyperventilators can spend years going from doctor to doctor seeking help.

"For the most part, physicians aren't trained to identify

habitual hyperventilators," says John H. Renner, M.D., a consumer health expert at Trinity Lutheran Hospital in Kansas City, Missouri. "A medical resident once described to me a patient complaining of 23 vague and seemingly unrelated symptoms. They were actually all symptoms of what we call 'chronic hyperventilation syndrome.' But the diagnosis never occurred to the resident because he hadn't been taught to look for it." Experts estimate that as many as one in every ten people who walk into a doctor's office are there because of chronic hyperventilation syndrome (CHS). Many mistakenly believe they have heart disease or a psychological disorder. Often, victims go through lengthy diagnostic workups with cardiologists, neurologists, psychologists, gastroenterologists, or allergists. Some never find out what's wrong with them. Others are branded hypochondriacs. "The worst thing that can happen is for the doctor to say, 'It's all in your head,' " says Dr. Renner, who has treated many of his own patients for CHS. "Symptoms of chronic hyperventilation syndrome are real."

He's not the only physician who believes that. Other physicians are piecing together the evidence and drawing similar conclusions.

Imitation Angina

Bernard Beitman, M.D., psychiatry professor at the University of Missouri School of Medicine in Columbia, points out that about 100,000 people with chest pain "pass" cardiac catheterizations each year. That means the test turns up no physical signs of narrowed coronary arteries, the main cause of angina pain. Yet, studies done six to ten years later show that 70 percent of these people continue to have chest pain, and 50 percent are disabled by their fear of heart attack.

So the question is, could CHS trigger angina-like chest pain?

"Cardiologists have said that there was some evidence that hyperventilation may cause spasms in the coronary arteries," Dr. Beitman says. "And coronary spasms could produce angina-like pain in the chest."

How is this possible?

Experts used to think that fast, shallow breathing did its mischief by robbing the body of needed oxygen. Now they know that hyperventilators inhale adequate oxygen, but they exhale too much carbon dioxide, an important metabolic regulator.

If your lungs throw off excessive carbon dioxide, your body becomes too acidic and a cascade of metabolic foul-ups follows. The smooth-muscle tissue lining blood vessels contracts, causing headaches or even chest pain. Your muscles may start to tire and cramp. Cells in your nervous system misfire, and you may feel dizzy or experience some tingling or numbness.

Of course, everyone's body reacts differently to the acid imbalance caused by CHS, so there's no way to predict which symptoms you might feel. But this finding does help to explain how symptoms of CHS might be mistaken for angina or even a heart attack. For most people, there's no easy way to tell the difference. So if you have the classic heart attack symptoms (chest pain, palpitations, shortness of breath, sweating, numbness, and tingling), assume it may be serious and get to a doctor or hospital.

Panic Disorder: Cause or Effect?

Unfortunately, the fear of suffering such symptoms sends some CHS victims into a state of panic—literally. Dr. Beitman interviewed 94 men and women whose cardiac catheterizations showed normal coronary arteries. Based on their answers, Dr. Beitman and his colleagues diagnosed 32 people (one-third of the group) as suffering from panic disorder, a type of anxiety reaction that in some patients may be caused by chronic hyperventilation.

Fast, shallow breathing is a signpost of panic attacks—those sudden, intense feelings of fearfulness with no obvious cause. Most physicians agree that people in the midst of a panic attack hyperventilate in response to the intense anxiety they feel. But now evidence suggests that, in some people, hyperventilation may actually precede the panic attack, triggering the kind of unfounded fears that typify such an attack. David H. Barlow, Ph.D., director of the center for stress and anxiety disorders at the State University of New York at Albany, estimates that hyperventilation is the primary problem in about one-half of panic-attack victims.

In these people, the very symptoms brought on by hyperventilation—light-headedness, dizziness, breathlessness—become a source of anxiety. This fearfulness then fuels the already-out-of-control breathing, which increases in intensity.

What Happens When You Hyperventilate?

Theories about how CHS gets started are as plentiful as the symptoms it can cause. Researchers at King's College School of Medicine and Dentistry in London report the most common causes include mild asthma, chronic bronchitis, protracted pain, anxiety, and depression.

Other experts say a lengthy period of high stress, like drawn-out divorce proceedings or financial problems, can start the hyperventilation habit, which stays after the problems are gone. Dr. Renner has seen a case of CHS start in a man who breathed lightly while his chest was taped to heal broken ribs. The breathing style that eased his pain remained after the tape was removed. Those prone to CHS may hyperventilate when they are tired or under stress, during or after exercise, while falling asleep or waking, or periodically throughout the day. This hyperventilation habit keeps carbon dioxide blood levels low, so CHS sufferers are always on the threshold of experiencing symptoms. Any normal increase in breathing—yawning, exercising, even laughter—can drop them into the danger zone.

Do *You* Hyperventilate?

It's not easy to tell if you're hyperventilating. To begin with, rapid breathing is a slippery symptom. "As soon as you focus on any automatic body function, like breathing, it's going to speed up," explains Dr. Barlow. So trying to time your normal breathing can backfire.

Shallow breathing, on the other hand, is simple to detect. If your breathing is too shallow, you'll notice that only your chest heaves when you inhale; your stomach doesn't move. Proper breathing expands your diaphragm (a kind of wall between lungs and stomach) to allow your lungs room to fill up with air, forcing your stomach to move, too.

To test yourself, lie down and place one hand on your chest and one on your stomach, just above your navel. If the hand on your stomach doesn't move at all while you inhale, you are breathing from your chest.

Of course, shallow breathing alone won't bring on chronic hyperventilation symptoms. You also have to breathe rapidly.

Other clues to CHS: Often you feel you are not getting enough air. You yawn or sigh a lot. When you are frightened, you hold your breath, then breathe out hard afterward.

There is a definitive CHS self-test, which Dr. Barlow describes in his how-to manual, *Mastery of Your Anxiety and Panic*. It involves consciously overbreathing to bring on the symptoms of hyperventilation. If you have unexplained symptoms (like chest pain, panicky feelings, dizziness, light-headedness, tingling in the fingers, chronic belching, or bloating) and they are indeed the result of CHS, the symptoms will appear during the test.

For safety's sake, however, don't attempt this test without a doctor's supervision. That is, ask to do it in his or her presence so he can monitor you. This is imperative, since people with heart disease and/or serious lung ailments like emphysema could suffer an adverse reaction.

If the test has uncovered a hyperventilation link, you can get on with treatment. Also, your doctor should know if you hyperventilate so he understands your symptoms and can check for possible related problems, such as cirrhosis, meningitis, or drug reactions.

Retrain Your Breathing

Based on evidence that some CHS symptoms arise because acid imbalance forces magnesium out of cells, researchers are investigating using magnesium infusions to control symptoms of CHS. But the current treatment of choice involves breath training.

Teaching yourself to breathe properly can take several weeks of exercises similar to the deep breathing taught in yoga classes. Dr. Barlow has developed this technique to help people suffering from anxiety, but he says it would help anyone who hyperventilates. (Note: Breathing retraining alone may not be enough for some people who suffer from panic attacks. You may need additional help from a qualified counselor.)

First, learn to breathe from your stomach. Lie face down on the floor with head sideways, resting on your cheek. Learn to push your stomach against the floor each time you inhale. Then, turn over and place a book on your stomach. Try to raise the book with each inhalation. If you habitually breathe from your chest, breathing from your stomach may make you feel like you're reeling out of control at first. Trust that you're in no danger and that the feeling will pass with practice. Once you've learned belly breathing, begin your practice sessions. Sit in a quiet, comfortable place and give yourself a few seconds to relax. Then, start counting your inhalations. Think "one" to yourself as you breathe in, then "relax" as you breathe out. "Two" in, "relax" out. Keep going until you reach ten, then return to one.

Repeat the counting sequence for 10 minutes twice a day, every day for one week. During this first phase of the program, don't try to change the speed or depth of your breathing. Breathing through your nose can help you resist the impulse to speed up. If you feel like you are not getting enough air, try pushing your stomach out just a little before you inhale.

During the second phase, start slowing your breathing by matching it to your counting. Say the number to yourself and then inhale. Think "relax" and then exhale. Then slow the counting rate a little each day until you are taking 10 breaths a minute. That would be inhaling for three seconds, then exhaling for three seconds.

You'll know you've reached the proper breathing rate when you can say "one thousand one, one thousand two, one thousand three" to yourself during one inhalation or exhalation. Check yourself occasionally with one hand on your chest and one on your stomach to make sure you're still breathing from your diaphragm. Practice for 10 minutes, twice a day for one week.

By the end of two weeks, you'll have learned to breathe properly in calm, quiet surroundings—even though initially just thinking about your breathing may make it speed up. Phase three calls for practicing your breathing technique throughout the day, at work, while shopping and especially in stressful situations. Each time, count from one to ten and back down to one again. Don't get discouraged if your technique doesn't go smoothly at first in real-life situations. You have the skill now, and you can get better with practice. After three weeks, you can continue the twice-a-day practice sessions, but it's important to remember to use the counting technique whenever you are under stress. Regular practice trains your lungs to breathe normally throughout the day.

CHAPTER 27

Is Your Iron High or Low?

By George L. Blackburn, M.D., Ph.D.

Don't pop supplements before getting your blood levels tested—and the facts straight.

Scientists have discovered the "irony of iron": Too many Americans aren't getting enough of it, and there's growing concern that a few are getting more than their bodies can stand. Either way there's trouble. Who are the people who need more? Who are the ones who need less? And how can you make sure your iron count is right on the mark?

For Lack of Iron

Everyone needs some iron. Many basic cell functions could not take place without iron, including blood production and the proper use of oxygen. If you don't get enough iron, your body can't produce enough red blood cells, which can lead to anemia. Symptoms of anemia include fatigue, weakness, pallor, and cold hands. It rarely causes death, but iron-deficiency anemia may be the world's most common disease, harming the quality of life of millions, especially in less-developed countries.

Iron deficiency also affects many people in this country. Who is most susceptible?

- Poor people, especially children, if their diets are inadequate.
- Menstruating women, who lose iron with each period. (Loss of blood means loss of iron.) They're particularly susceptible if they don't eat much food because they are watching their weight. It's been estimated that iron deficiency occurs in a third to half of healthy, young American women.
- Pregnant and lactating women. Pregnancy, childbirth, and nursing take a large toll on iron levels, so most pregnant women and new mothers need iron supplements (after checking with their doctors, of course).
- A small percentage of African-Americans who have a hereditary problem called sickle-cell anemia. They may be slightly more susceptible to an iron deficiency because their iron absorption is reduced.
- Men or women suffering from heavy bleeding for any reason.
- The ill or frail elderly. They're more likely to be iron deficient (and also more likely to lack in other key nutrients) than their healthy peers.

If you're in one of these risk groups, you should talk to your doctor about whether you might benefit from iron supplementation. A routine and inexpensive blood test that gauges your iron can tell the tale. If you're not in one of these groups and you eat a reasonably diverse diet, it's likely that you're consuming enough iron to meet your needs.

Iron Overload

Doctors used to think that iron overload was very rare, and we would routinely prescribe iron supplements to many patients. Now we're thinking twice.

Iron overload is usually not caused by eating too many iron-rich foods. Instead, it is triggered by a combination of factors: first, a genetic propensity and, second, years of overdoses of iron from repeated blood transfusions or iron supplementation.

The body stores iron in the liver. The danger is, if levels go too high, they can overload and harm the liver, conditions referred to as hemosiderosis (iron overload) and hemochromatosis (overload to the point of damage). Symptoms of these disorders include bronzing of the skin, diabetes, enlarged heart, heart arrhythmias, loss of libido, abdominal pain, and arthritis. Hemosiderosis used to be quite rare, but in recent years scientists have found that it is increasingly prevalent and that cases may be aggravated by iron supplementation.

Not everyone is susceptible to iron overload. People have different abilities to absorb iron. Caucasians of Northern European extraction may be the most susceptible. A small but significant number of them carry a gene that allows for absorption of too much iron. Early studies had indicated that this tendency was quite rare, but now it's estimated that about 2 to 3 per 1,000 people in the United States may carry this genetic susceptibility. Up to 10 percent of Caucasians of Northern European extraction are at risk.

Remember, even if a person is genetically susceptible, overload to the point of physical damage takes years of high doses of iron.

If you're in one of the deficiency risk groups we mentioned, you probably don't need to worry about iron overload. If you're not taking iron supplements, it's also unlikely to be a problem. But if you are a healthy man or nonmenstruating woman and also a Caucasian of Northern European extraction, you should be wary of prolonged iron supplementation. No one should take an iron supplement without having their blood iron levels tested first. Don't assume it's safe without that testing and a doctor's okay.

The Iron-Rich Diet

The best way to avoid either iron overload or iron deficiency is to eat a healthy, balanced diet, with a diversity of nutrient-rich foods. If you get enough iron from foods, you probably won't need supplements.

Since iron deficiency is a far more common problem than iron overload, it's important for most people to eat iron-rich foods. Lean meat is the best source of iron. Part of the reason is that the iron in meat is in a form that's easy for the body to absorb. Modest servings of low-fat meats should be eaten several times a week.

Although many vegetables contain iron, the amount our bodies can absorb varies because of other chemical compounds present in vegetables. A Swedish study indicates that good iron absorption results from consumption of carrots, potatoes, beets, pumpkin, broccoli, tomatoes, cauliflower, cabbage, turnips, and sauerkraut. (These vegetables all contain ascorbic acid, malic acid, or citric acid, which enhance absorption.) On the other hand, some vegetables that contain a lot of iron can't really provide most of it to our bodies because they also contain a lot of phytate (a compound that blocks absorption). These not-too-good sources of iron include butter beans, lentils, beet greens, and, believe it or not (sorry, Popeye), spinach.

CHAPTER 28
Sail
through Menopause

A host of tips to help diminish hot flashes, heavy periods, and more.

For generations, women anticipated menopause as they would an impending storm. They braced themselves, hoped to be spared the worst of it, then sat tight until it passed. Now, finally, that attitude is dissipating.

"We know that estrogen withdrawal at menopause leads to changes all over the body, including the brain," says Boston gynecologist Isaac Schiff, M.D. The physical and emotional ramifications of these changes are well known. But they're also quite variable. The fact is, for most women, menopause passes like a gentle wind rather than a hurricane-force gust. In a five-year study of nearly 2,500 women who went through menopause, 85 percent of those asked about symptoms said they are never depressed.

Still, we cannot forget that the hormonal shifts of the menopausal years do have the power to disrupt some lives. And there is deepening concern that, as estrogen wanes, heart disease and osteoporosis become major threats to all women. But, now, thanks to a better understanding of the menopausal process, we can take action to counter the assault.

The Withdrawal Process

Strictly speaking, a woman reaches menopause on the date of her very last period, usually by age 50 or 51. But, because estrogen production declines gradually—and periods can be "missed" before they actually stop—you can't be sure you've passed menopause until you've been period-free for an entire year. At this point, you know the ovaries' estrogen production has dropped too low to stimulate the endometrial lining of the uterus in preparation for pregnancy.

Of course, the menopausal years stretch far beyond this point, in both directions. Many women first notice their bodies changing during their forties. And the physical and emotional changes can last up to ten years after their last period. In fact, for many women the menopausal years will account for up to one-third of their lives.

Hot Flashes and "Night Sweats"

Perhaps the most universal menopause symptom is hot flashes. Seventy-five percent of women experience them. Thankfully for most, they occur less than once a day, are mildly annoying and subside after a year or so. But hot flashes can be tormenting. They can strike in rapid succession, just 10 to 30 minutes apart, or arouse you from your sleep in the middle of the night. Many experts say that these "night sweats" are to blame for the irritability so many menopausal women feel. What's worse, some women may continue having hot flashes for five years or more.

The research into hot flashes is relatively new, but a few clues to the biological mechanisms involved have emerged. Estrogen influences the production of neurotransmitters, which carry messages to and from the brain. So, as estrogen dwindles, the brain's relay system may go awry. As a result, blood vessels may suddenly dilate, increasing circulation to the face and neck; at the same time, the body's thermostatic control may go out of kilter, bringing on the flush of heat characteristic of a hot flash.

What can you do to avert a strike or lessen the impact?

Keep a log. Note the date, time, intensity, and duration of the hot flash. Also, record the circumstances preceding it: what you ate or drank, how you felt emotionally.

After you've logged several episodes, try to identify any patterns. You may find, for example, that your hot flashes are more severe when you drink alcohol, which dilates blood vessels. Or, perhaps they hit harder when your emotions heat up. In a six-week study of ten menopausal women, psychologist Linda R. Gannon, Ph.D., found that, for half of the participants, stress was associated with increased frequency, intensity, and duration of hot flashes.

Try biofeedback. This technique, which uses electronic sensors to detect changes in body temperature and muscle tension, has helped many migraine sufferers stifle their headaches. And, at least in this case, what halts a headache may help a hot flash.

Through feedback from the sensors, people learn what it takes to consciously relax their facial muscles and warm their hands (achieved by conjuring up mental images of, say, basking in the sun). Barry L. Gruber, Ph.D., a Washington, D.C., psychologist, uses biofeedback to train patients in relaxation, hand cooling, or hand warming. For some women biofeedback doesn't work, he says, but others do seem to be able to cool hot flashes with the technique.

To find a qualified biofeedback center nearest you, Dr. Gruber suggests that you contact the Biofeedback Certification Institute, 10200 West Forty-fourth Avenue, Suite 304, Wheat Ridge, CO 80033; (303) 420-2902.

Or try hypnosis. A hypnotic technique helped some women reduce the intensity and length of hot flashes in a small study conducted by Malkah Notman, M.D., psychiatry professor at Harvard Medical School.

In hypnosis, the woman is helped to relax with the

guidance of a qualified professional. The suggestion is then made for the woman to think of a cool scene such as a mountain stream. She's taught how to use this experience on her own, and can return to this state to initiate a sensation of coolness when she feels a hot flash coming on. This technique, though, doesn't work for everyone.

To explore this option, ask your physician to recommend a qualified professional or health center that offers hypnosis for quitting smoking or reducing tension. Then call and inquire if the staff will work with you on hot flashes.

Cool off. Slip off your sweater, sip a cool drink, switch on the air-conditioner. Anything that helps cool you off on a sultry summer day will relieve a hormone-triggered heat wave. Just be prepared to rewarm yourself a few minutes later, says Dr. Schiff; hot flashes are often followed by strong chills.

Incidentally, as a bedtime preventive against night sweats, soak in a tepid tub till the water cools or lower the thermostat to about 60 degrees before you turn in. One of Dr. Gannon's subjects had a ceiling fan mounted over her side of the bed with a switch at hand.

Don't fight it; relax. Your impulse may be to panic or tense up as the sensation overtakes you. Instead, stop what you're doing, sit down and just let your arms and legs hang loose. Imagine the waves of heat passing freely over you. All the experts we spoke with suggested you may be able to lessen the intensity of a hot flash by changing how you think about it.

Evaluate the possible benefits of vitamin E. Lila E. Nachtigall, M.D., New York University gynecology professor, says 400 international units of vitamin E taken twice a day can cut the frequency of hot flashes for some women. Do check with your physician before beginning vitamin E supplementation, however. While the vitamin is generally considered safe, it can have a blood-thinning effect.

Consider hormone-replacement therapy. Hormone treatment is considered the most effective treatment for debilitating hot flashes that do not respond to self-care remedies. Discuss this with your doctor (see "HRT: The Pros and Cons" on page 241).

Heavy Periods

As the ovaries' estrogen production begins to fluctuate, in the early stages of menopause, menstrual periods change. Many women are relieved to find their menstrual flow getting lighter. Others may miss periods for a few months, only to face a period that is heavier than ever. What can you do?

See your doctor. Though common in the menopausal years, heavy menstrual bleeding can have serious ramifications. Periods that are exceptionally heavy or last much longer than usual can put you at risk of iron-deficiency anemia. Of even greater concern, any heavy bleeding that occurs after you've gone one year period-free could be a warning sign of cancer.

Eat lots of iron-rich foods. To counter iron deficiency, look to lean beef and beans, your best dietary sources of iron. Or, if blood tests have determined that you are indeed anemic, consider iron supplements.

Avoid alcohol. Alcohol dilates the blood vessels. And although it can't cause a heavy period, it can exacerbate the problem, says Kathleen MacPherson, R.N., Ph.D., researcher at the University of South Maine, in Portland.

Beware of substances that may thin your blood. Certain medications, including aspirin, can interfere with the blood's clotting ability. Vitamin E has blood-thinning side effects as well. Ask your doctor or pharmacist for guidance.

Ease off strenuous exercise. Even if you're accustomed to heavy workouts, it may be too fatiguing during a heavy period, says Dr. MacPherson. Mild exercise, like leisurely walking, is fine if you feel up to it. But postpone more strenuous activities like high-impact aerobics.

Consider hormone-replacement therapy. The hormone progestin can put an end to heavy flow. Your doctor may want to try progestin if a heavy period persists and he has performed the necessary tests to make sure your uterus is healthy.

Vaginal Symptoms

Like other menopausal effects, vaginal changes are individual: sudden and severe in some women and so gradual they practically go unnoticed in others. When estrogen is withdrawn, vaginal walls may become thinner and lose moisture, making them more vulnerable to irritation. Some women report itching and burning; intercourse may cause bleeding and pain. Menopausal hormone changes also disrupt the delicate pH of the vagina, creating a hospitable environment for yeast and bacterial infections. At the same time, the muscles supporting the vagina, uterus, and bladder may become lax.

But don't get discouraged. While vaginal changes may be inevitable to a certain extent, they don't have to become troublesome if you follow these suggestions.

Choose personal hygiene products with care. Use mild (nondeodorant and fragrance-free) soap or cleansing bars. Avoid personal hygiene sprays, which can irritate dry, sensitive vaginal tissues.

Dry thoroughly after a shower or bath. If your perineal area remains damp, bacteria could multiply and invade vulnerable vaginal tissues. To be safe, use a blow dryer on a cool (not hot) setting to remove excess moisture between your legs. Also, always wear cotton-crotch pantyhose and underwear. Cotton "breathes" better than nylon, allowing moisture to evaporate.

Think twice about using antihistamines. Antihistamines don't discriminate; they dry mucous membranes in the nose and in the vagina. If you need to treat an allergy or nagging cold, ask your pharmacist or your doctor to suggest an alternative medication.

Strengthen pelvic muscles. Specially designed Kegel exercises zero in on crucial muscles: Use the same motion you would to stop a stream of urine to contract the pelvic muscle. Do 10 contractions a day: five fast, plus five held for three to five seconds. Build up to a total of 50 or 100 contractions a day.

Keep sex alive. Regular sexual activity helps keep natural moisture flowing and maintains pelvic muscle tone. Gloria A. Bachmann, M.D., gynecology professor at Robert Wood Johnson Medical School in New Brunswick, New Jersey, recommends that women indulge in a relaxing, warm (not hot) bath before sex to relieve tension arising from meddlesome menopausal symptoms. And don't forget birth control. No matter how erratic your menstrual cycles, you're not pregnancy-safe until you've put an entire year between you and your last period.

Replace lost lubrication. If dryness becomes a problem, you may want to try a brand-new nonprescription lubricant, called Replens. It comes in single-dose, tamponlike dispensers, used every three days to provide continuous lubrication. Dr. Bachmann and a colleague tested Replens on 89 menopausal women who said the product stayed in place better than a standard water-soluble lubricant applied with a dispenser. Another advantage: The lubricant helps normalize vaginal acidity, thus reducing the risk of infections. One note of caution: If you have a history of allergic reactions to medications, use this product only under a doctor's care.

Consider hormone-replacement therapy. Experts say that even the most severe vaginal symptoms can be reversed with estrogen in doses lower than are needed to resolve hot flashes. Sometimes, too, estrogen cream applied directly to the vagina can alleviate the itching and dryness with fewer potential side effects than oral estrogen. Discuss hormone options with your doctor.

Depression

The good news is some research suggests that many women don't get the so-called menopause blues. What's more, it seems that some menopausal women who are depressed are likely to have had a history of depression before they entered menopause.

That's not to belittle the blues in those who do succumb. An emotional challenge arises from the "symbol" of menopause, says Dr. Gannon. Hot flashes and vaginal symptoms are unmistakable messages from your body that it's growing older. This, and the central fact of menopause— loss of the ability to bear children—demands an emotional adjustment even in this day of expanded lifestyle opportunities for women.

If these issues get the best of you, consider the following suggestions.

Encourage mutual support among your peers. Dr. Gannon says any activity, from church socials to political fund-raising events, that brings you together with other women your age will help. "When people are isolated, they tend to feel their problems are unique," says Dr. Gannon. "It's a relief to find out that other women feel the same way they do." If you can't locate a group, don't fret. A Friend Indeed newsletter provides a forum for menopausal women's concerns. (For a free introductory copy, send a self-addressed, stamped envelope to: A Friend Indeed Publications, Inc., Box 515, Place du Parc Station, Montreal, Canada H2W 2P1.)

Take a brisk walk. Evidence suggests that regular, energetic exercise may improve your mood by raising levels of endorphins (circulating good-humor hormones known to drop during menopause).

Seek professional counseling. Dr. Gannon says you should get professional help if you feel so low you can't get out of bed in the morning or you no longer have the will or ability to lift your spirits on your own. Ask your physician to recommend a qualified therapist. Some mental health specialists set their fee according to a sliding scale based on what you can afford to pay for treatment. And treatment is increasingly covered by insurance.

Irritability and Other Mental Disturbances

When nighttime hot flashes disrupt sleep, women understandably become fatigued and irritable, says Dr. Gannon.

But women can cope with these mental disturbances. Here's how:

Walk, bike, or join an aerobics class. Aerobic exercise enhances blood flow to the brain, improving thought processes. You'll also feel more energetic and benefit from the companionship, says Dr. Gannon. A recent study showed that regular aerobic exercise made middle-agers more satisfied with their shape and appearance—two measures of self-esteem that suffer during menopause.

Schedule fatigue-fighting sessions. If your irritability is caused by sleepless nights, take an afternoon nap or a morning meditation break. Sit quietly with eyes closed.

Let your muscles go limp, breathe slowly, and repeat a single word to yourself. When other thoughts intrude, don't shove them out of your consciousness. Just let go of them gently and return your attention to the word you're repeating. Practice for 10 to 20 minutes, each day.

Keep your sense of humor. Hot flashes may not be your idea of a joke, but learning to laugh at them may reduce the anxiety they can cause, says Dr. Gannon. As an example, one of her patients jokes that she's getting her money's worth out of her perfume now that her hot-flash-warmed skin radiates the scent.

Find a sympathetic doctor. A doctor who's willing to answer your questions and explain the physical changes you're undergoing can ease your anxiety. "If your doctor takes a high-handed approach to discussing menopause, or pooh-poohs your concerns, it's time to look elsewhere," says gynecologist Wulf H. Utian, M.D., a founder of the North American Menopause Society (NAMS). The society currently lists more than 300 qualified physicians. For the doctor nearest you, write to NAMS, 29001 Cedar Road, Suite 600, Lynhurst, OH 44124.

Say no to dizzying sedatives. Older people were more likely to suffer a hip-fracturing fall while on long-lasting tranquilizers in a study at Vanderbilt University School of Medicine in Nashville. Ask your doctor about alternatives.

Consider hormone-replacement therapy. Estrogen replacement therapy can't resolve personal problems, but it can relieve the anxiety caused by hot flashes and other physical discomforts. (It can't, however, relieve depression.) An understanding doctor can help you evaluate whether your distress warrants a trial with hormones.

Strengthening Your Heart

While changes that menopause brings to your body and psyche can be annoying and disruptive, its long-term effect on your cardiovascular system can be life-threatening. Heart disease and stroke are the biggest cause of death for women over age 40.

The connection between menopause and heart disease seems to lie in estrogen's ability to keep women's levels of artery-clogging blood fats lower than their male partners', says Frank M. Sacks, M.D., Harvard Medical School researcher. As women stop pumping out estrogen, they lose their hormonal advantage.

In a study at the University of Pittsburgh, researchers measured cholesterol levels in 101 women ages 42 to 50 before and after they'd hit menopause. One-third of the menopausal women were given estrogen replacement therapy; their cholesterol levels remained unchanged. But the menopausal women who did not receive estrogen had notable changes in their cholesterol. Specifically, their levels of high-density lipoproteins (HDL)—the so-called good cholesterol that protects against disease—decreased and their low-density lipoproteins (LDL)—the "bad" cholesterol—increased. The researchers conclude that changes in cholesterol caused by menopause add to the increase in heart disease risk that is caused by aging.

Dr. Sacks recommends women use the same diet and exercise techniques that men do to blunt heart disease risk factors. For example:

Stop smoking now! Your gain will be twofold: You'll escape from a known heart-damaging habit and possibly postpone menopause itself. Studies show that smokers begin menopause earlier than nonsmokers do, although no one knows exactly why.

Take a 30- to 40-minute walk every day. In one year, sedentary women in a British study lowered their total cholesterol and raised the good HDL component by walking for about 2½ hours a week at a brisk pace.

Relax. Do yoga. Practice meditation. Take time to play. Dean Ornish, M.D., director of the Preventive Medicine Research Institute in Sausalito, California, suggests that regular relaxation sessions may help slow your body's production of artery-obstructing cholesterol.

Eat a low-fat, high-fiber diet. Focus your diet on high-fiber fruits, vegetables, grains, and beans with lean meats, fish, and dairy products. Fatty foods (especially those that are high in saturated fat and cholesterol) can send your blood cholesterol sky high. Plus, fatty foods are the major dietary contributor to fat on your frame. And being overweight can tax your cardiovascular system, too.

Rate your heart disease risk. Have your doctor evaluate your cardiovascular status so you know what you're up against. Have your blood pressure and cholesterol levels checked and a blood sugar test for diabetes, a known risk factor for heart disease that becomes more common in older people.

Consider hormone-replacement therapy. Estrogen's ability to improve cholesterol levels—raising the good HDLs and lowering the bad LDLs—is one reason doctors prescribe it for postmenopausal women who are at high risk for heart disease.

Building Strong Bones

Like heart disease, osteoporosis—the bone-thinning disease—threatens the quality of your life after menopause. The Achilles' heel of osteoporosis is the hip joint: two-thirds of postmenopausal women whose weakened hips fracture never regain full mobility. In fact, their risk of dying increases in the six months following the break.

There's no way to turn back the clock on bone-depleted skeletons. Building bone throughout life is your best chance for fighting osteoporosis. But by taking the following steps during menopause, you can help reduce your risk:

Keep your calcium intake high. Your body requires a steady supply of calcium to keep bones strong. Though the U.S. Recommended Daily Allowance for menopausal women is 800 milligrams, some experts recommend 1,200 milligrams daily to be on the safe side. Choose two or three calcium-plus foods each day: low-fat milk and milk products, broccoli, kale, sardines, mackerel, and tofu.

Weather permitting, get outside for a brisk walk each day. Nothing beats weight-bearing exercise—that's the type needed to help keep bones intact. Walking is perfect. And, in just 15 minutes of outdoor exercise, you'll soak up enough of the sunshine vitamin (vitamin D) to help strengthen many of your bones.

Try gardening, swimming, or tennis. Researchers have found that staying involved in a wide range of exercises sharpens women's sense of balance. So they may avoid

HRT: The Pros and Cons

Hormone-replacement therapy (HRT) can improve the quality of life for some menopausal women. By reducing the risk of heart disease and osteoporosis, it may even save lives. But before you decide, consider:

- Studies have established that taking estrogen alone for more than two years significantly increases a woman's risk of endometrial cancer (cancer of the lining of the uterus). Taking low doses of estrogen with progestin, however, appears to negate this risk.
- There is some concern that HRT is linked to breast cancer. While the link is far from conclusive, physicians recommend that women with a history of breast cancer proceed with caution. Also, to be on the safe side, all women should be advised to have a mammogram prior to HRT, to rule out existing cancer, and yearly while taking hormones.
- HRT is not recommended to women who smoke, due to increased risk of blood clots and stroke.
- Ask your physician about the potential risks and benefits of HRT so you can decide on your best course of treatment.

falls or cushion the crunch by catching themselves when they tumble.

Consider hormone-replacement therapy. Hormones can hold off osteoporosis for as long as you take them. If your doctor decides you're at high risk, a test called bone densitometry can tell you how dense your bones are, and how much you can afford to lose.

CHAPTER 29

The Ups and Downs of Estrogen Therapy

Physicians agree that hormone-replacement therapy is a very personal decision.

It's a high-stakes decision, a woman's choice of whether to go on hormone-replacement therapy at menopause. Indeed, the potential benefits are significant: Estrogen-replacement therapy begun at menopause can not only relieve debilitating hot flashes and vaginal atrophy, but also prevent osteoporosis, the thinning of bones that causes fractures (some of which, in older women, can be life threatening). And research has raised the tantalizing probability that estrogen wards off heart disease, the number one killer of American women.

But nagging concerns over possible health risks, including cancer, have cast a shadow over the use of estrogen.

"It's not so much that hormone-replacement therapy is controversial," says Elizabeth Barrett-Connor, M.D., chair of the Department of Community and Family Medicine at the University of California, San Diego. "It's that there are a lot of unanswered questions."

Understandably, women contemplating estrogen therapy are in a quandary. To help guide those of you making this very important decision, here's what you need to know before you say yes—or no.

The Bright Side

Hormone-replacement therapy (HRT) usually involves a regular program of estrogen, to replace the natural estrogen that wanes at menopause. Sometimes, another hormone, progesterone (typically progestin, a synthetic form), is added to the estrogen regimen. The hormones are available in pills, though sometimes they're administered through creams, skin patches, or vaginal suppositories. Millions of menopausal and postmenopausal American women are now on HRT, and some physicians say many more could benefit from the treatment. Their reasons are primarily threefold:

1. Estrogen-replacement therapy can improve menopausal symptoms by as much as 95 percent. With the decline of estrogen, about 25 percent of women experience insomnia, hot flashes, and vaginal atrophy. For some, the symptoms are severe; sexual intercourse may be virtually impossible.
2. Estrogen treatment begun at menopause is considered the best preventive treatment available for osteoporosis. Bone density dwindles rapidly after menopause. The result can be debilitating fractures. But if estrogen treatment is begun at or immediately after menopause, it minimizes that bone loss, for as long as a woman stays on the hormone.
3. Studies suggest that estrogen-replacement therapy prevents heart disease in postmenopausal women. "Heart disease is the most common cause of death in older women," says Dr. Barrett-Connor. "If those studies are confirmed, this could be the biggest single benefit for estrogen-replacement therapy." Meir Stampfer, M.D., a Harvard scientist who has studied estrogen's cardio-protective effect, says that the data are nearly conclusive. For reasons not fully understood, he says, estrogens affect cholesterol levels. They usually raise the good high-density lipoproteins (HDLs) while lowering the bad low-density lipoproteins (LDLs).

A Link to Breast Cancer?

But even physicians who are convinced of estrogen's heart benefits have reservations about its use. "The ultimate and unanswerable question concerns the breast cancer/ estrogen connection," says William Castelli, M.D., medical director of the Framingham Heart Study. It is known that most breast cancers are estrogen dependent; that means

The Nonhormonal Alternatives

To reduce hot flashes: There are other drugs, besides hormones, to control hot flashes and other menopausal symptoms. Talk to your physician. Natural remedies are worth trying, too. Lila E. Nachtigall, M.D., associate professor of gynecology at New York University, recommends 400 international units of vitamin E twice a day for hot flashes. "In some cases, this vitamin therapy decreases the number of flashes," she says.

For sexual health: Water-soluble lubricants can remedy vaginal dryness. Regular sexual activity with a partner or alone, and Kegel exercises, also help keep the vagina toned. Kegel exercises involve contracting and releasing the same muscles you use to stop urine flow. Begin by squeezing tightly, hold for a few seconds and then relax. Do these daily, working up to 50 to 100 contractions a day.

To combat osteoporosis: The American College of Obstetricians and Gynecologists suggests postmenopausal women who are not on estrogen take 1,500 milligrams of calcium a day. Frequent weight-bearing exercise, such as walking, also helps keep bones strong. Cigarettes and alcohol take a toll on bones and increase likelihood of fracture. Of course, calcium and exercise help the most if they are begun before menopause. They're not as effective as estrogen in stopping bone loss after menopause.

There are other drugs being used on a limited basis to combat bone thinning. Physicians have high hopes for a new class of drugs called diphosphonates, which are being tested in the United States and used in Europe.

"Diphosphonates have exactly the same effect on bone as estrogen, but without stimulatory effects on the reproductive system. It's entirely investigational, but I'm confident they will be widely available soon," says Dr. Riggs.

To promote heart health: Relax. Take a 30- to 40-minute walk every day. Eat a low-fat, low-cholesterol, high-fiber diet. Lose any excess weight. And, if you smoke, quit. These are a few of the many ways, besides hormones, to lower cholesterol and heart disease risk.

For beauty: Some women want estrogen for its widely rumored—but scientifically unproven—cosmetic effects. "This is not a reason to go on estrogen," says Patricia Barwig, M.D., a gynecologist in Milwaukee, Wisconsin. "Many glamour/fashion magazines say estrogen improves your skin. But I think not smoking, staying out of the sun, using adequate moisturizers, and drinking a lot of water does more for your skin."

---

estrogen fuels their growth. So, in a woman with an existing, undetected (and possibly dormant) breast cancer, estrogen could conceivably accelerate the cancer's growth, says Lila E. Nachtigall, M.D., associate professor of gynecology at New York University.

Whether estrogen therapy actually increases breast cancer rates in women who take it after menopause is still a subject of debate. Some studies confirm a link; others refute it. Many experts characterize the medical evidence as confusing.

In the final analysis, even the widely publicized Swedish study (published in the *New England Journal of Medicine*), seems to have created more questions than it answered.

The largest, longest-term study to examine the effect of hormone therapy on breast cancer rates, the Swedish effort followed more than 23,000 HRT users for up to nine years and longer. The study found estrogen use increased a woman's risk of breast cancer by 10 percent. And the longer a woman used the drug, the higher the risk. Women with more than nine years of estrogen use were 70 percent more likely to develop breast cancer than normal.

Physicians point out, however, that the majority of participants in the Swedish study took a form of estrogen called estradiol, which is more potent than the "conjugated estrogens" prescribed to most Americans. Conjugated estrogens may be safer than estradiol, they say.

In fact, 22 percent of the participants did use conjugated estrogens, and researchers found no increased risk of breast cancer among them. As reassuring as that sounds, American physicians remain cautious.

The actual number of women on conjugated estrogen was relatively small, they say. And few of them took the hormones for more than five years. So we don't know the long-term effect.

And so, we await further research to clarify this issue.

On the Uterine Cancer Risk

Meanwhile, studies have established that taking estrogen alone for more than two years significantly increases a woman's risk of endometrial cancer (cancer of the uterine lining).

Estrogen doesn't actually cause uterine cancer. But it can push a dormant or precancerous endometrial condition over the edge into a full-blown cancer. "And the longer you take estrogen, the greater the risk of this," says George R. Huggins, M.D., chairman of the gynecology department at the Francis Scott Key Medical Center in Baltimore.

To eliminate the risk, physicians prescribe lower doses of estrogen combined with progestin. The incidence of endometrial cancer in women on estrogen/progestin regimens is even below that of women who get no hormone treatment at all.

The Potential Pitfalls of Progestin

Sounds like progestin is a healthy addition to HRT. But now new questions are being raised about its safety, too.

"It used to be thought that progestin might prevent the development of breast cancer," says Isaac Schiff, M.D., chief of the Vincent Gynecology Service at Massachusetts General Hospital, Boston. "Now we're leaning away from that. We know that progesterone stimulates breast tissue, we have to be open to the possibility that it promotes breast cancer," Dr. Schiff says.

Indeed, in the Swedish study cited above, breast cancer risk was highest among women who took estrogen with progestin for long periods. The combination hormone therapy increased the risk of breast cancer more than fourfold after six years. But again, this is far from conclusive, since the number of participants who took this combination hormone treatment was very small. More research is needed. Another concern is that progestin reduces the heart-protecting benefits of estrogen. Progestin has the opposite effect of estrogen on blood lipids; it lowers good HDLs and raises bad LDLs.

"The use of progestin definitely reduces the benefits of estrogen for lipid profile," says Dr. Stampfer. "If women take progestin, they may well be undoing part or most of the heart benefit of estrogen, though we don't know this for sure." The combination of estrogen and progestin, and the lower doses, were not used widely in the United States until the 1980s. So the long-term consequences are simply not known.

What's a Woman to Do?

Until the uncertainties are resolved—which won't be for years—how do you decide whether HRT is for you?

Every physician we spoke with agreed the decision is very personal. "Each woman has to decide for herself based on the current available information," says gynecologist Mitchell Levine, M.D., of Cambridge, Massachusetts. After talking with leading physicians and looking at the research, we can offer these suggestions.

Find a concerned, well-qualified physician to expertly guide you. A good doctor not only can help you make the big decision (whether or not to begin hormone-replacement therapy) but also can help you find the right type and dose of hormones to maximize benefits and minimize side effects and risks. Throughout your treatment, stay in very close touch with your physician, for both monitoring and new information. "There is no substitute for a good gynecologist to work with you," says Dr. Castelli.

Always consider your alternatives to hormone therapy first. "There are many ways to reduce the risk of heart disease," says Dr. Stampfer. "Taking estrogen is one. But there are other good ways, such as diet and exercise, that don't involve the risk." Similarly, lifestyle changes (especially if begun before menopause) can provide adequate protection against osteoporosis for most women. Moderately troublesome hot flashes and other menopausal symptoms may respond to nonhormonal treatments as well. (See "The Nonhormonal Alternatives" on page 244.) HRT should be prescribed only when menopausal symptoms are very severe, says Dr. Nachtigall.

If you're taking hormones primarily to relieve vaginal symptoms, try hormone creams or suppositories. The local application of hormone creams carries fewer overall health risks than the ingestion of hormone pills.

If you have a personal or family history of estrogen-dependent breast cancer, it's prudent to avoid HRT. Or at least proceed with extreme caution and careful medical supervision. Admittedly, the final verdict on the HRT–breast cancer link isn't in yet. But given the fact that a woman with a family history of breast cancer has a higher-than-average chance of developing the disease, many physicians interviewed said they'd be reluctant to prescribe HRT.

If you have a history of blood clotting or strokes—and, especially, if you are a heavy smoker—avoid HRT. Studies have shown that birth-control pills that contain high doses of estrogen encourage strokes and thrombophlebitis (blood clots in veins). HRT with low-dose estrogen does not seem to have the same effect. In fact, some research suggests estrogen-replacement therapy may actually protect against strokes and clotting. Nonetheless, Dr. Castelli, a renowned cardiovascular specialist, said he'd be reluctant to prescribe estrogen to anyone with a history of clotting or strokes. "And if she's a heavy smoker, I definitely would not recommend she go on postmenopausal estrogen," says Dr. Castelli. "The combination of smoking and estrogen may encourage clotting."

In addition, if you suffer from fibroids or endometriosis (estrogen fuels both conditions), liver disease, migraines, gallbladder disease, or seizure disorders, you may be well advised to avoid hormone therapy. Daughters of women who took diethylstilbestrol (DES) during pregnancy may have reproductive changes that may make use of estrogens dangerous.

If you've had a hysterectomy and oophorectomy (removal of the ovaries), estrogen therapy may offer some benefits. Symptoms of estrogen withdrawal can be particularly severe following an early surgical menopause. And with the uterus removed, endometrial cancer, a major drawback of estrogen therapy, is no longer a worry. Since you don't need progestin to ward off endometrial cancer, it may be best to avoid it. Discuss this with your physician.

If you have a family history or are otherwise at high risk for osteoporosis, HRT may protect you. If there's a consensus among physicians, it's that the women who can most clearly benefit from HRT include those at high risk for osteoporosis. But keep in mind, most women are not at risk for severe osteoporosis. To confirm your risk at the time of menopause, get a bone scan of the lumbar spine, says B. Lawrence Riggs, M.D., vice-president of the National Osteoporosis Foundation. (Ideally these noninvasive tests should be done at a reputable medical institution.

Get a mammogram before you begin HRT. Hormone therapy may accelerate the growth of cancerous breast tumors. And mammography is the only way to detect early, unpalpable breast cancers.

Closely monitor your breasts during hormone treatment. "I tell patients that though there is no strong evidence that estrogen in modest doses for postmenopausal women causes breast cancer, we have to keep our eyes and ears open all the time," says Dr. Schiff. To be on the safe side, have a mammogram once a year, a breast examination by a physician twice a year, and practice breast self-exam every month.

If you're taking estrogen without progestin (and you haven't had a hysterectomy), schedule an annual endometrial biopsy. Endometrial cancer associated with estrogen use has a high cure rate, if it's detected early. And, according to the American College of Obstetricians and Gynecologists, with regular endometrial biopsies (an office procedure), precancerous conditions can be caught and treated before a full-blown cancer even develops. Unfortunately, endometrial biopsies can be uncomfortable and, sometimes, painful. But, in this situation, they're an absolute necessity; they could save your life.

Another important note: Report any abnormal bleeding to your physician immediately; it can be a warning sign of uterine cancer.

Keep tabs on your cholesterol. Blood fats, including cholesterol, should be checked, then monitored annually to determine the effect of estrogen and/or progestin, says Leon Speroff, M.D., professor of obstetrics and gynecology at the Oregon Health Sciences University.

If you have a history of hypertension, monitor your blood pressure closely. Another long-held concern is that estrogen could exacerbate high blood pressure. With lower doses, some physicians say, this is not the case. "Estrogen usually lowers blood pressure," asserts Rogerio Lobo, M.D., chief of reproductive endocrinology at the University of Southern California School of Medicine, Los Angeles. "Still, about 5 percent of women taking estrogen will develop hypertension."

Take the lowest-dose hormones for the shortest period possible. Long years of estrogen therapy may increase your risk of endometrial and breast cancers, among other health problems.

For safety's sake, it's best to use the lowest effective dose for the shortest amount of time possible. (For HRT, 0.625 mg of conjugated estrogen is considered a low dose.) Some menopausal symptoms may temporarily return when you discontinue hormone treatment, though gradual reduction of estrogen minimizes this effect. To stave off osteoporosis, some experts say, the longer you take estrogen, the better. "Most of the data suggest you do get large bone losses when you stop estrogen therapy, and the rate of loss is similar to the rate of loss following menopause," says Dr. Riggs.

Nevertheless, several other physicians told us they believe that even shorter-term estrogen therapy may be an osteoporosis benefit. "In theory, if you could delay bone loss for 10 years, it's an advantage," says Dr. Barrett-Connor. "I'm uncomfortable giving estrogen for more than 15 years because we don't know the long-term effects."

(For more information, read "Taking Hormones and Women's Health: Choices, Risks and Benefits," a booklet by the National Women's Health Network, available for $5 from the National Women's Health Network, 1325 G

The Hassles of HRT

Estrogen and progestin do cause some women unpleasant, though not dangerous, side effects. Some women who begin estrogen report breast tenderness, nausea, headaches, psychological changes, and weight gain. Dr. Huggins says that estrogen may take a bad rap on the last charge, weight gain. "Postmenopausal women who don't take estrogen have just as much difficulty controlling their weight as women who do," he says.

Progestin is far more likely than estrogen to cause unpleasant side effects, physicians say. Given together with estrogen, progestin may cause regular vaginal bleeding similar to a monthly period. In addition, "about 25 to 30 percent of women experience depression, oily skin, temporary weight gain, headaches, or leg cramps—all the premenstrual kinds of symptoms—as a result of taking progestin," says Dr. Huggins. Reducing the dose and altering the type of hormones you're taking can help minimize the side effects. In some cases, doctors prescribe natural progesterone, administered through vaginal suppositories, which may be better tolerated than progestin.

Street NW, Washington, DC 20005, and *Estrogen: The Facts Can Change Your Life*, by Lila E. Nachtigall, M.D., and Joan Rattner Heilman, published by Price/Stern/Sloan, Inc., Los Angeles, and available in paperback for $6.95.)

CHAPTER 30

Pap Test Update

Everything you need to know about the test every woman needs.

Most women take this relatively simple cervical cancer screening test for granted as a basic part of self-care. And with good reason. Since its development in the 1940s by George Papanicolaou, M.D. (hence the test's name), deaths from cervical cancer have plummeted more than 70 percent. On the other hand, the American Cancer Society (ACS) recorded 7,000 U.S. cervical cancer deaths in 1988. Most women who develop cervical cancer have not had regular Pap tests.

But the test has become the focus of controversy. Various professional organizations have fought over ideal Pap test frequency, and error rates estimated as high as 50 percent have tarnished the test's once-spotless reputation.

Because of these controversies, many women have lost faith in the Pap test at the very time it's most necessary. Alarming increases in cervical cancer have been reported in other countries. And in the United States, many physicians are seeing larger numbers of abnormal Pap tests in younger women—even teens. Many authorities believe the rise in cervical cancer is due to the spread of the human papillomavirus (HPV), which causes venereal warts. Scientists now think HPV may also cause cervical cancer as well.

All this presents a very confusing picture. Once viewed as a simple preventive health measure, the Pap test has become a source of anxiety and apprehension. Fortunately, the haze is beginning to clear. Both the government and the medical community are taking steps to ensure accuracy. The papillomavirus is being studied more closely. And authorities have reached consensus about Pap test frequency. Nonetheless, women themselves must still take responsibility for ensuring the accuracy of their tests.

The cervix is the neck of the uterus. Shaped like a tiny doughnut, it protrudes into the back of the vagina. The cervix may develop three types of cancer—squamous cell, adenocarcinoma, and adenosquamous—and the Pap test can detect all three, but it is best at detecting squamous-cell cancer, the most common type. It can also occasionally pick up infections and vaginal and uterine cancers. But its primary purpose is to detect cervical cancer and its precursors.

Cervical cancer usually has no symptoms. Occasionally, a woman with the disease may notice spotting, bleeding, or vaginal discharge. But cervical cancer is generally painless and may remain undetected for several years. It usually grows slowly, but studies indicate that certain types may progress rapidly.

The ACS estimates that nearly 13,000 new cases of invasive (spreading) cervical cancer appeared in 1988. But early cervical cancer is far more common. An estimated 1 to 4 percent of women have cervical dysplasia, an abnormality which may progress to cervical cancer. If detected in its early stages, cure rates top 90 percent, but early diagnosis is critical.

Who Is at Risk?

Until recently, cervical cancer was very rare in women under 25. But over the past decade teenagers have begun to show surprisingly high rates of cervical dysplasia and even cancer.

Scientists presume this trend is linked to increasing sexual activity among teenagers. Cervical cancer is now thought to be a sexually transmitted disease linked to the human papillomavirus. Cervical cancer is almost unheard of among groups such as Roman Catholic nuns, who abstain from sexual intercourse. And risk increases in direct

Human Papillomavirus and Cervical Cancer

Human papillomavirus (HPV) is the sexually transmitted cause of venereal warts (condylomata). These warts may appear on the cervix, the vulva, a man's penis or scrotum, or in or around the anus. Previously, scientists believed warts were benign, and treated them conservatively. However, in the past few years, research has linked HPV to cervical cancer.

Researchers once suspected the herpes virus as a contributor to cervical cancer, but recently attention has shifted to HPV. This virus has been found in up to 95 percent of cervical cancers. It alters cell functions in ways that suggest it causes cancer. And women infected with HPV appear much more likely to develop cervical dysplasia.

Not all studies agree about HPV's role. Only a few of the 40 types of HPV have been associated with cervical cancer. And an association with cancer doesn't necessarily mean HPV causes the disease. Many risk factors contribute. But women infected with HPV carry a significantly increased risk for cervical cancer. And the incidence of HPV is increasing, especially among teens. Because it is sexually transmitted, scientists attribute at least part of the increase in HPV to increased sexual activity.

HPV is a treatable illness, best caught before it has a chance to transform cervical cells to dysplasia. After treatment for HPV, a woman should be monitored more closely by her clinician because she is still at higher risk for cervical cancer. The fact that HPV can be detected by the Pap test is another reason to have regular exams.

But prevention is important as well. Practitioners have found that cervical cancer is less likely among condom or diaphragm users. And they recommend limiting the number of sexual partners and refraining from casual sex or encounters with those who have multiple sex partners.

Margarita Lengyel, M.D., an Akron obstetrician and gynecologist, also believes in treating the partner. "I ask all my HPV patients to have their partners checked for venereal warts. I tell them that until both are free of warts they should use condoms."

proportion to women's—or their lovers'—number of sexual partners.

Another important risk factor is lack of—or irregular—Pap screening. Women who have never had Pap tests have about five times the average risk, and women who haven't had a Pap test in the last five years have a threefold increased risk.

Other cervical cancer risk factors include cigarette smoking and birth control pills. Cervical cancer is 2½ times more likely in heavy smokers than in nonsmokers. Women who use oral contraceptives for more than five years face 1½ times the average risk.

Interpreting Results

Pap tests gather cells from the transformational zone (T-zone) of the cervix, where most cancers occur. (The T-zone is so named because during fetal development, the area contains columnar cells that later become transformed into mature squamous cells.) To locate the cervix, the clinician inserts a speculum, an instrument shaped like a duck's bill with hinges. Then using a cotton swab (or small brush) and a wooden spatula, the clinician collects three samples of cells from the cervix's T-zone, places them on slides, and sends them to the lab for analysis.

A Pap test should not feel painful. Tell your clinician if you experience any pain during the exam.

The ideal time for a Pap test is 12 to 14 days after the start of your last period. To ensure accuracy, don't douche before the exam, and avoid vaginal medications and hygiene products.

Though effective, the Pap test is merely a screening test. It can point to probable cancer or precancer, but it cannot give a definitive diagnosis.

Cervical cancer develops in stages, and Pap tests are graded that way, though in reality one stage merges gradually into the next. To understand the grading system, some terms must be defined:

Cervical metaplasia means that mature surface cells extend down into cervical tissue, a normal process that takes place in the cervix's T-zone. This is *not* cancer or precancer.

Cervical dysplasia means some abnormal cells are present. Cervical dysplasia is *not* cancer. However, if left untreated, it may progress to cervical cancer.

Cervical Intraepithelial Neoplasia (CIN) means "new growth"—an abnormal number of immature rapidly dividing cells. The epithelium is the layer of "skin" cells that line the cervix, similar to the lining of the mouth.

The new system for interpreting Pap smears is by CIN classes. Possible Pap test results include:

Normal. The cells collected are healthy, flat, mature cervical cells with tiny nuclei. There are no immature cells.

Metaplasia. Some cells in the sample reflect the normal transformation processes of the cervix, while others don't. The unusual cells show no precancerous changes. This is *not* an abnormal test result.

Infection or inflammation. Bacteria, white blood cells, and some immature cells appear in the sample. The clinician may begin treatment if the test indicates an infection. Occasionally, Pap test results may be unclear because of infection. If so, the clinician should repeat the Pap test after the infection resolves.

CIN I. Abnormal potentially precancerous (dysplastic) cells are growing on the cervix. The number of these immature, rapidly dividing cells is small and limited to about one-third of the epithelial layer. Although dysplasia is *not* cancer, the cells may eventually become cancerous. The clinician may conduct further tests to determine the extent of abnormality.

CIN II. The sample shows a larger percentage of immature cells. At this stage, the growth is still small, occupying about two-thirds of the epithelium, but hasn't penetrated deeper. Again, the clinician may conduct further studies.

CIN III. At this stage, all or most of the slide cells are immature. This implies that the growth of abnormal cells occupies the full thickness of the epithelium. CIN III is also known as *carcinoma in situ*, cancer that is confined to one location. It can usually be removed without danger of further spreading.

Suspect microinvasive or invasive cancer. Abnormal cells may have penetrated beyond the cervix's epithelial layer. However, depending on the degree of penetration, even invasive cancers have a fairly good prognosis when treated promptly.

Treatments

Only about 2 percent of Pap smears show CIN or invasive cancer. And of those women with abnormal tests, the large majority are curable. But cervical cancer starts with only a few cells. Over time, the disease can spread. The key is early diagnosis and treatment.

Clinicians treat inflammatory Pap tests with antibiotics appropriate to the infection and usually follow treatment with an additional Pap test.

Controversy surrounds treatment for early dysplasia (CIN I). Some clinicians take a wait-and-see approach and repeat the test after a few months because CIN I may resolve without treatment. Others take a more aggressive approach and treat all stages of dysplasia. They fear a repeat Pap test may give a false negative result—a "normal" while the woman still has CIN I—and delay treatment.

Margarita Lengyel, M.D., former chief resident of Obstetrics and Gynecology at Akron General Medical Center in Ohio and now an Akron area obstetrician/gynecologist, favors the more aggressive approach. "Any kind of dysplastic cells warrant colposcopy," she says. "That's the fairest thing for women with CIN I."

Most clinicians agree that CIN II, CIN III, and invasive cancer should be treated aggressively. The specific treatment depends on a number of factors including the stage of the disease and the individual woman (e.g., age, other health conditions, desire for continued fertility, etc.).

Since the Pap test is only a screening test, a positive result tells the clinician to take a closer look. The most likely follow-up tests after abnormal Pap tests include:

Colposcopy. Colposcopy allows close examination of the cervix. A colposcope is similar to a pair of binoculars. The doctor looks through the instrument after applying a special stain to the cervix to highlight abnormal areas. The clinician may take tissue samples (biopsies) of these areas and send them to the lab for closer analysis.

Colposcopy is painless. However, if the clinician needs to take a biopsy, you may experience spotting and cramping afterward. After biopsy, avoid tampons, douching, and intercourse for at least a week to allow the cervix to heal.

Endocervical curettage (ECC). Often performed along with colposcopy, the clinician places a small spoon-shaped scraping device inside the cervical canal to sample cells in that area. This relatively painless test allows the clinician to check the entire cervix.

According to Dr. Lengyel, "The doctor should always do an endocervical curettage because the canal is one area you can't see. If you don't sample the endocervix, you're not doing a complete colposcopy."

Conization. This type of biopsy is both a treatment and diagnostic test. In cases where the clinician is uncertain of the diagnosis, or where CIN extends beyond the view of the colposcope, conization allows removal of the abnormal tissue. Conization may also be used for women with severe dysplasia (CIN III) who might be treated with hysterectomy, but who wish to remain fertile.

Performed in a hospital under general anesthesia, the surgeon makes a circular incision in the lining of the outer cervix and then removes a cone-shaped piece of tissue that extends into the cervical canal and removes the entire cervical lining. If lab analysis shows the clinician removed the entire abnormality, no further treatment is necessary. But if the tissue doesn't contain all of the abnormality, the woman requires more therapy.

Conization poses many possible complications so it's generally not recommended as a primary therapy. Heavy bleeding may require transfusion. Scarring may impair fertilization or impede menstrual flow. And poor cervical functioning (cervical incompetence) may result in premature delivery during pregnancy.

For women with definitive diagnoses, or with less-advanced CIN, simpler treatments are available. If the CIN is within view of the colposcope, treatment options include:

Electrocautery. The physician uses an electrical probe to kill the abnormal surface cells. The procedure can be performed in the doctor's office and may cause pain for a few seconds. After the abnormal cells die, healthy cells replace them.

Cryosurgery. The doctor destroys abnormal cells with a probe supercooled with nitrous oxide or carbon dioxide. This technique is usually less painful than electrocautery, but mild cramping is common. Compared with electrocautery, cryosurgery causes less bleeding and involves less risk of cervical blockage (stenosis), but the woman usually experiences a heavy vaginal discharge for up to six weeks following the procedure.

Laser therapy. The clinician uses a high-energy beam of light to vaporize abnormal cervical cells. A precise treatment performed in the hospital with either local or general anesthesia, it results in little or no vaginal discharge and less scarring than other techniques. But it requires a skilled clinician with specialized training. It also costs about five times as much as other procedures.

"For CIN I and II," says Dr. Lengyel, "you can offer the woman cryosurgery. For anything beyond that, laser surgery is probably the way to go. Cryosurgery and laser therapy are equally effective for slight to moderate dysplasia (CIN I and II). Cryosurgery is cheaper, the woman doesn't need general anesthesia, there's not that much discomfort, and it's just as effective."

Hysterectomy. Hysterectomy may be an option for severe CIN or invasive cancer.

Close follow-up is essential for women who've undergone cautery, cryosurgery, conization, or laser therapy. Frequent Pap tests confirm that treatments were effective,

How Often?

For years most physicians and all the major medical organizations recommended annual Pap tests for all women over 18 and for younger women who were sexually active. Then, a few years ago, following the lead of British and Canadian authorities, the American Cancer Society (ACS) broke ranks and recommended Pap smears only once every three years following two normal annual screenings. The revised recommendations drew heated protests, particularly from the American College of Obstetricians and Gynecologists (ACOG), whose spokespeople insisted the yearly Pap test and annual pelvic and breast exams were the only way to go. The American Medical Association (AMA) also joined the fray on the side of ACOG, calling for a return to the annual Pap test. Meanwhile, women were left confused about how often they should be tested.

The ACS recommendation was based on a 1976 Canadian study. A second Canadian study performed in 1984 suggested more frequent exams were indeed safer.

In 1987, the warring organizations reached a compromise. The ACS, AMA, ACOG, the National Cancer Institute, the American Academy of Family Physicians, the American Nurses Association, and the American Medical Women's Association all adopted this recommendation: "All women who are or have been sexually active, or have reached the age of 18 should have an annual Pap test and pelvic examination. After three or more consecutive satisfactory, normal exams, the Pap test may be performed less frequently, at the physician's discretion."

Margarita Lengyel, M.D., an Akron obstetrician and gynecologist, says she continues to conduct annual exams even after several consecutive normal exams. "I recommend a yearly Pap test. A Pap test isn't expensive, and it isn't painful, so I think it's best to have it annually, especially today with the increasing incidence of venereal warts. Sometimes Pap tests are negative a couple of times, then suddenly turn positive with moderate dysplasia or cervical cancer. That scares me. I think the yearly exam is the best way to go." She also recommends Paplike cell sampling for women who have had hysterectomies to check for vaginal cancer.

In the new guidelines, the phrase, "are or have been sexually active, or have reached the age of 18" is particularly important. It reflects new awareness of the rise in dysplasia—and even early cancer—in girls 15 to 19.

Postmenopausal women should continue to have annual Pap tests. Older women are at significant risk for cervical cancer, accounting for 25 percent of U.S. cases.

Although the controversy has officially ended, clinicians still differ on Pap test frequency recommendations. If you feel your Pap tests are performed too infrequently or too often, discuss your concerns with your clinician. Both of you need to feel comfortable with the decision.

and alert the woman and her clinician to any renewed CIN. Success rates for cautery, cryotherapy, and laser therapy are all 90 percent or higher when the disease is treated promptly.

CHAPTER 31

Say Good-Bye
to Varicose Veins

Today, virtually all spider and small varicose veins can be removed quickly and painlessly without surgery.

Many people deal with varicose veins or the smaller, "spider" veins the same way: They just cover up their legs and silently rue the problem. What other options are there, outside of major surgery?

The answer: more than you think.

"Unfortunately, the surgical stripping of the body's longest veins (the saphenous veins), which run from the groin to the ankle, is still being done routinely and far too often at most community hospitals," says John Bergan, M.D., one of the nation's foremost vascular surgeons. "But now, leading doctors are advocating a less radical, much more cosmetic, very selective procedure for treating problem veins."

Unsightly
and Uncomfortable

At least 10 percent of American men and 40 percent of women are troubled by varicose veins—those bumpy bluish veins that, in the worst scenario, resemble bunches of grapes. Many more have spider veins—the tiny, blue or red veins often found in weblike clusters on the thigh.

Varicose veins develop when valves that run the length of the saphenous vein give out, trapping blood in the lower extremities. When this happens, weakened areas of vein walls bulge under the pressure of the excess blood.

Genetics seems to play a key role; some people may have a natural weakness in their vein walls. Hormones, too, may contribute to their development; many women develop varicose veins during pregnancy presumably because heightened hormone levels weaken vein walls.

Superficial spider veins can be caused by trauma, such as being smacked by a tennis ball. But usually, they are very tiny offshoots of underlying varicose veins, says California dermatologist Mitchel Goldman, M.D. "I use the analogy of varicose veins being your arm, and spider veins being your fingers." Fortunately, neither is considered a serious medical problem. But varicose veins and, to a lesser extent, spider veins can cause nagging symptoms: aching, heaviness, and fatigue in the legs; itching; muscle cramps at night. These symptoms tend to worsen during the menstrual period.

The good news is that now the cure won't leave scars as unsightly as the varicose veins themselves.

Treatment by Injection

Today, virtually all spider veins and smaller varicose veins can be removed quickly and painlessly through a nonsurgical technique called sclerotherapy.

The concept of sclerotherapy is simple: A solution—usually saline or sodium tetradecyl sulfate—is injected into the vein. The solution irritates the vein, causing it to collapse and eventually dissolve. Zap!

Sclerotherapy isn't new. It's been around as long as the hypodermic needle, some 130 years. But side effects, such as skin ulceration, have tarnished its image. Today, safer solutions, finer needles, and improved techniques have brought sclerotherapy back in favor. In a survey of 200 people who have undergone the procedure (mostly for spider veins), 98 percent expressed satisfaction with the outcome.

The procedure takes 15 to 45 minutes per session. Treatment usually involves a series of at least three to four sessions, spaced over several weeks. The cost of the sclerotherapy varies widely among doctors. Medical insurance often does not cover it.

Also, you should be aware that sclerotherapy still has some side effects. Your leg may be swollen and bruised, possibly for several months, following the procedure, says Dr. Goldman. And 5 to 30 percent of those who have sclerotherapy will develop brown pigment or freckling on the skin. This freckling is usually temporary, Dr. Goldman explains, but in some cases, it can last up to two years. (This side effect is more likely to occur in people who are extremely overweight.) Keep in mind, too, that sclerotherapy is not a cure for unsightly veins since new ones can crop up. Many doctors recommend that patients wear compression stockings continuously for a few hours to several weeks after therapy. Compressing the area is believed to help keep new varicose or spider veins from forming. Even so, some people may need a yearly sclerotherapy touch-up.

"Sclerotherapy is like taking care of cavities," says Walter de Groot, M.D., F.A.C.S., a surgeon in Seattle. "When your dentist says you're through, he doesn't mean you're never going to see him again. He just means you're done for now."

Outpatient Surgery

Despite the obvious appeal of a nonsurgical procedure like sclerotherapy, some varicose veins are simply too large to be closed by injection. Dr. Bergan, for one, believes that varicose veins larger than 3 to 4 millimeters (over $\frac{1}{10}$ inch) in diameter probably require surgery for long-lasting results. He and other leading surgeons, however, believe that most people can benefit from a modified surgical technique that removes only defective segments of the saphenous vein rather than the entire vein.

"With the traditional surgery, if a woman had 17 varicose

Go Easy on Your Veins

Doctors say there is no way to prevent spider or varicose veins. But excess weight and inactivity—as well as having a job in which you stand or sit a lot—can all increase pressure in the legs and aggravate problem veins. To minimize the symptoms and prevent mild problems from getting worse, try these tips:

- Wear support hose. In fact, doctors recommend them if you're pregnant or have a job where you sit or stand a lot—whether or not you have varicose veins. They can improve circulation and reduce achiness.
- Give your legs a lift. Raise your legs above hip level to ease discomfort. Or, better yet, combine the powers of gravity and support hose in the following exercise: Slip on your support hose. Then lie flat on your back, raise your legs straight up in the air, resting them against a wall. Hold this position for two minutes.
- Repeat throughout the day, as often as needed. This allows the blood to flow out of the swollen leg veins back toward the heart.
- Take off excess weight. Extra pounds put unnecessary pressure on your legs.
- Don't smoke. A report from the Framingham Heart Study noted a correlation between smoking and the incidence of varicose veins. The researchers concluded that smoking may be a risk factor for those with a predisposition to varicose veins.
- Walk! There's nothing better to improve the health of your legs. It improves circulation and prevents pooling of blood by strengthening the calf muscle that pumps blood up the leg toward the heart.

veins, when she woke up afterward she had 17 scars," says Dr. de Groot, who is also president of the North American Society of Phlebology (vein specialists). "In most cases, with the new technique, a single inconspicuous incision is made in the crease of the groin. In rare, severe cases, an additional incision is made at the knee." Other incisions, if necessary, are so tiny they don't even require stitches.

There's more to recommend it, too. It requires only a local anesthetic, which reduces the surgical risk over the older method. You usually don't have to stay in the hospital overnight. And, compared to sclerotherapy, the incidence of recurrence is about half as likely after five years, according to Dr. Bergan.

Fortunately, the older, stripping method is on its way out; 56,000 were done in 1982 compared to 33,000 in 1987, the last year for which figures are available, according to the National Center for Health Statistics.

Still, for some people, only the traditional surgery will do. "It seems to depend entirely on the extent to which the saphenous veins are incompetent," says D. Eugene Strandness, Jr., M.D., professor of surgery at the University of Washington School of Medicine. But the good news is "We now have better techniques to identify the saphenous veins that are not working than we did before," says George Johnson, Jr., M.D., chief of the section of vascular surgery at the University of North Carolina in Chapel Hill.

A bewildering array of physicians treat vein problems—vascular surgeons, plastic surgeons, general surgeons, dermatologists, internists. But finding a competent doctor trained in sclerotherapy or the latest surgical techniques may take some work on your part. No medical or government board certifies this field.

The trouble is "not too many doctors are devoted to vein diseases because they're not considered serious medical problems," says J. Leonel Villavicencio, M.D., director of the Venous and Lymphatic Surgical Clinic at Walter Reed Army Medical Center. "Even vascular surgeons tend to prefer arterial surgery [such as bypasses] to vein surgery and may not be trained properly in venous disease."

Generally, however, vascular surgeons do handle advanced cases of varicose veins. Plastic surgeons usually deal with the relatively uncommon spider veins on the face (the only area where the oft-ballyhooed laser is now a useful treatment).

Your family doctor, dermatologist, or internist can help you locate a qualified specialist. Then, when you make the appointment, be prepared to ask a lot of questions. Inquire about the doctor's success rate and complication rate. Ask him how much experience he has had with the procedure. "I'd want them to have been doing it at least once or twice a week for a couple of years," says Dr. Goldman. Also, try to speak to a couple of patients who have undergone the same treatment with the physician. Remember, the treatments described above are only as effective as the physician who's performing them.

CHAPTER 32

Spot-Reduction Weight Loss: At Last

Though not a substitute for diet and exercise, liposuction does wonders on bulges you just can't budge.

"I exercise and I eat right. I really work hard to keep myself in shape."

That's why it seemed so unfair to 51-year-old Jan Etheredge that the little pouch of fat on her belly wouldn't budge. Neither sit-ups nor serious dieting fazed it.

"It bugged me for years, and when I finally had the chance to have it removed, I thought, 'Why not? What have I got to lose—besides this darned potbelly?' "

Two months later, in a cosmetic surgeon's office, the

California grandmother had the fat on her lower abdomen sucked out, in a procedure called liposuction. Today, she says, she has the flat stomach she's yearned for. Her only reminder of the operation is a ¼-inch scar hidden just below the pubic hairline.

Jan Etheredge's experience is an example of liposuction at its best. Today's most popular cosmetic surgery, liposuction offers a no-sweat solution to certain stubborn fat deposits. And there's a bonus: "When fat is sucked away, it's gone for good," says William Coleman, M.D., a dermatologic surgeon. As an adult, you can no longer produce new fat cells to replace those removed. Excess calories will have to be stored elsewhere.

Appealing? You bet. But don't forget, liposuction is a surgical procedure with all the complications and health risks that go along with that. And, as more than a few people will attest, there's a chance you won't achieve cosmetically acceptable results. Proceed with caution. Before you submit, get the facts and, most important, make sure you're in good hands.

How It's Done

To perform liposuction, a doctor inserts a blunt-ended metal tube, called a cannula, through a small incision in the skin, then tunnels repeatedly under the skin in a radiating pattern to dislodge and remove fatty tissue. The cannula is connected by a plastic hose to a vacuum aspirator, which suctions out the fat, which is mingled with blood and body fluids.

The procedure can be done under local or general anesthesia. Usually, an intravenous line drips a glucose solution into your arm during the 30 to 90 minutes it takes for the surgery.

Afterward, you must wear support garments, such as a girdle or chin strap, depending on the liposuction site, for a few weeks. This helps prevent dimpling by smoothing out the fat that remains under your skin. If your thighs, buttocks, or hips are suctioned, you may not be able to walk or sit comfortably for a few days. Bruising, swelling, and some pain may linger for up to three months. "Should you develop a fever, report it to your doctor. It could indicate an infection," says Texas surgeon Howard Tobin, M.D. "This is a very rare complication but it's one of the more worrisome."

The cost is anywhere from $1,500 to $6,000, depending on where you live and the extent of the surgery. Also, liposuctions performed in a hospital may cost considerably more than those done in a doctor's office. Expect to pay in full in advance. In most cases, medical insurers do not reimburse for this procedure.

Who's Likely to Benefit?

Even if you can afford it, liposuction may not be for you. Contrary to popular belief, it's not for weight watchers seeking an alternative to dieting and exercise. In fact, doctors discourage seriously overweight patients from this procedure unless there is an associated medical problem, such as chafing thighs or a constant yeast infection under a fold of fat.

That's because liposuction is a form of surgical spot reduction; no more than five pints of aspirated material should be removed at one time (and even that's a lot). Also, the more fat you've got, the more skin you have encasing it. When the fat's removed, the skin may sag. A face-lift or tummy tuck can take up the slack, but combining liposuction with yet another surgical procedure increases risk.

While doctors admit a younger patient usually makes a better liposuction candidate, age per se isn't so much a consideration as overall health and skin tone. Skin that's sun damaged or otherwise thin and lax won't spring back into shape after liposuction. Without a follow-up scalpel assist, the results are often unacceptable: sagging or drooping skin.

The best candidate is a healthy person of average weight with taut, resilient skin—and a person who, like Jan Etheredge, has a specific bulge to resolve (see "Is Liposuction for You?" on page 270). Liposuction is most effective in reducing those genetically doomed, diet-and-exercise-resistant fatty pockets on the hips, thighs, stomach, waist, or chin. Calves and ankles, however, pose tricky problems.

Is Liposuction for You?

While there are no hard-and-fast rules for success, here are some general guidelines to consider.
You're an excellent candidate if you . . .

- Maintain good health
- Are at your ideal weight
- Are age 40 or younger
- Have excellent skin tone (pinch the skin on the back of your hand; if the skin snaps back the moment you let go, your skin has good tone)
- Do not have a history of bleeding tendencies.

You're an average candidate if you . . .

- Maintain good health
- Weigh no more than 10 pounds above your ideal weight
- Are between ages 40 and 60
- Have somewhat resilient skin

You're a poor candidate if you . . .

- Weigh more than 20 pounds above your ideal weight
- Are age 60 or older
- Have thin or lax skin (pinch the skin on the back of your hand; if your skin doesn't snap back when you let go, your skin tone is lax)
- Smoke
- Have diabetes, cardiovascular disease, phlebitis, or a metabolic disorder.

Because the blood supply to these areas isn't as good as to the rest of the body, there's a much higher risk of infection.

Choosing Doctor Right

Of course, "for optimum cosmetic results with minimal complications, the most critical factor is who performs the liposuction," says R. Barrett Noone, M.D., a plastic surgeon from Philadelphia. Look for a physician who is well trained to do this procedure and is equipped to handle a life-threatening emergency, should one arise.

Plastic surgeons, cosmetic surgeons, dermatologic surgeons, dermatologists, and other physicians all perform liposuctions. Many plastic surgeons contend they alone are qualified; prospective patients should seek physicians certified by the American Board of Plastic and Reconstructive Surgery, they say. The advantage of this, explains Dr. Noone, is that you can be sure your physician has been fully trained to handle surgical emergencies.

Of course, dermatologists and other doctors who do liposuction note that surgical emergencies are extremely rare and that they are just as qualified as plastic surgeons to perform the procedure. In fact, as Dr. Coleman points out, some hospitals offer dermatology residents more liposuction training than plastic surgery residents.

If you're having a large area or multiple areas done—or if you need a skin tuck along with liposuction—look for a physician who's experienced in handling similar cases.

Unfortunately, though, because liposuction has become so popular (and lucrative for physicians), it's lured many unqualified practitioners. And that's a major concern. Any doctor can set up shop, advertise, and perform liposuction with no training at all.

That's why it's so important to ascertain your physician's competency with this procedure. Ask him or her the following questions:

- Are you board-certified, and by what board? To make sure it's one of the 23 boards approved by the American Board of Medical Specialties, consult the ABMS Compendium of Certified Specialists at your public library or

Suck Away Cellulite?

Liposuction can't smooth out areas of cottage-cheese-textured fat on thighs and buttocks, often referred to as cellulite. But a new procedure that's similar to liposuction, called cellulite-release surgery, can reduce dimpling, says Julius Newman, M.D., of Philadelphia, founder of the American Society of Liposuction Surgery.

The lumpy appearance of cellulite occurs because fat bulges out around long, tough fibers of tissue that stretch from muscles (beneath the fat) to the skin. In cellulite-release surgery, usually the doctor first aspirates the fat (through a standard liposuction technique). Then he inserts a ¼-inch-wide forked instrument through the small incision in the skin. The instrument has rounded tips to prevent it from puncturing the skin. It also has a cutting edge at its center, which catches and severs the fibers that are causing the dimpled skin. The doctor makes many passes with this instrument, in a radiating pattern.

So far, Dr. Newman has performed cellulite-release surgery on about 60 patients. "People with extremely bad cellulite can expect only fair results," he says. "But those with mild cellulite have excellent results." None of his patients experienced complications.

Cellulite reduction is so new that few doctors or medical associations have heard of it, much less formed an opinion about it. Currently, only a few physicians nationwide are performing cellulite reduction. Like any new medical procedure, your best bet is to wait to see if it develops a good track record before seeking it for yourself.

contact the American Board of Medical Specialties at
(312) 491-9091.

- Do you have hospital surgical privileges, or, at least, hospital admitting privileges, and where? Surgical privileges mean a doctor has been reviewed by his peers and accepted into the medical community at that particular hospital. Admitting privileges have less weight, though it does mean that you can be admitted if a complication occurs.

- If you do liposuction in your office or at an outpatient facility, is the facility accredited, and by what organization? The major accrediting organization is the Accreditation Association for Ambulatory Health Care. Accreditation means the facility meets standards similar to a hospital operating room for cleanliness and emergency equipment. Unfortunately, very few nonhospital facilities are accredited. That doesn't necessarily mean they're not acceptable. But it does mean you should consider all other factors carefully.

- Do you carry liability insurance? Doctors who operate out of their offices are not required to do so.

- Can I speak with a few of your patients who've undergone liposuction? Call them.

Then, as a final check, call your local medical society to find out if complaints have been filed against the doctor. Remember, your results depend, more than anything else, on your doctor's skill.

CHAPTER 33

Fuzz Busters

By Pamela Boyer

Prevention *magazine's beauty editor shares the lessons she learned when searching for pain-free electrolysis.*

I'd often toyed with the idea of electrolysis. But I had been hesitant to try it because of the time and expense required, and because of the possibilities that the hair would grow back and the procedure would leave scars. My biggest fear was that it would hurt.

My concerns were bolstered by an article I read by a doctor who had decided to try electrolysis, since he recommended the procedure to his patients. The outcome didn't sound encouraging. He went to two different technicians and found one "unbearably painful."

I'd also heard differing descriptions from other people who'd tried electrolysis, from "I practically fell asleep during the treatment," to "It just about killed me." Despite the daunting reports, I decided I really should find out for myself.

A Slow Start

Because electrolysis requires a series of treatments, I wanted to find a local electrologist. And because there are no national standards regulating the profession, and some states don't even require electrologists to be licensed, I reasoned that a physician's recommendation would improve my chances of finding a qualified practitioner.

I contacted local gynecologists, dermatologists, and endocrinologists. Surprisingly, of the 12 doctors I called, less than half could refer me to an electrologist. Worse, none of these referrals were recommendations. Instead, I was

told, "Here's the name of an electrologist we've sent patients to in the past and we've had no complaints."

If at First
You Don't Succeed . . .

When I arrived, the electrologist explained the process and
equipment and took a brief medical history.

Electrologists use several variations on two main types
of electrolysis (permanent removal of hair at least partly
using electricity). The older type is galvanic, using electricity to convert body salts to lye to kill a hair root. The other
main type, thermolysis, kills the hair root by converting
electricity into heat. The first electrologist I met combined
the two procedures.

This electrologist also explained that hair goes through
three phases: The first is active growth. In the second, the
resting phase, the hair stays in the follicle as it dies. In the
third phase, the hair follicle becomes dormant and the
dead hair falls out. Electrolysis is effective only on hairs in
the growing phase. Dormant follicles need to be zapped
again, because when the dead hair falls out a new hair will
take its place.

At my first session, I was given damp, felt-covered han-
dles to hold in both hands. Each handle was connected to
the electrolysis machine, which means my body was acting
as the electrical ground. The electrolysis needle was
attached by a wire to the machine. Surprisingly, the part
I was most afraid of—the insertion of the needle—wasn't
even uncomfortable. After the needle was in the hair follicle, the electrologist released a charge of electricity to fuse
the fluids in the follicle and kill the root. The jolt did
hurt—but not unbearably. It ranged from the traditional
mosquito-bite description to that of a hornet sting.

The electrologist then lifted the dead hair out with tweez-
ers. Sometimes the hair didn't release freely, which meant
that the root wasn't totally destroyed and the hair would
regrow.

I seemed to feel the current more during the second
treatment, which took place a week later. After each treatment the skin beneath my brows became pink and tender.

The electrologist explained that the small bumps caused by my skin's reaction to the heat of the needle are fairly common. They go away within a day or so. I'd suggest you schedule your appointment at a time when you won't be out in public immediately afterward.

On my next two visits the discomfort seemed to get progressively worse—fewer mosquito bites and more hornet stings. At its worst, the pain made my eyes water. On my third visit I had to ask that the treatment be stopped after only 10 minutes of what should have been a 15-minute appointment.

I found out later why the process may have been so painful. Some operators use the needle inaccurately, zapping both follicles and bare skin. Some apply the needle longer to hair roots that didn't die after the first application. And often in subsequent treatments, some operators simply get sloppier.

. . . Try, Try Again

I didn't want to quit, however. I decided to try a different electrologist. She used the same equipment but the treatments were less painful. Still, after four treatments I had much more regrowth than I'd been led to expect. The results were partial at best and there seemed no end in sight. Although I felt discouraged, I decided to try once more. This time I went to Lucy Peters, International, an electrology group recommended by a dermatologist in Philadelphia, where Peters has one of her treatment centers.

Prices were not as expensive as I'd feared. Locally, electrolysis cost between $30 and $40 per half-hour visit. Lucy Peters, International, charges $50 per half hour, the minimum length of a session.

Before my session I visited Lucy Peters in her quiet Manhattan offices. We talked about electrolysis in general and the equipment she has helped develop. She is thoroughly knowledgeable.

Peters introduced me to the technician who would be working with me. My operator, Terri, took a detailed account of my current health status and medical history to be sure I had no preexisting medical conditions, such as wearing a pacemaker, which would rule out electrolysis.

The next step was to decide exactly how I wanted my eyebrows to look. Neither of the other electrologists had done this. While I looked in a magnifying mirror, we discussed my natural brow line. Peters is adamant about having the end result look natural. "After all, electrolysis is permanent," she said. "If you want to experiment with trendy styles, do it by tweezing. Your permanent shape should suit your face."

Once we'd agreed on how much should be taken out and where, Terri took a "before" photo of my eyebrows for their records and for me to compare to the end result.

Expertly Equipped

The treatment lasted about half an hour, but I could have gone longer! The treatment itself caused only occasional, minor discomfort. Lucy Peters attributes this success to both the specialized equipment she uses and to the intensive training that her operators receive.

"We use an insulated bulbous probe instead of a needle, and we developed the LPS 1118 Epilator to deliver the current necessary to destroy the hair on the first try.

"The insulated probe prevents the current from destroying anything but the bottom portion of the hair, which is the only part that grows. The skin itself is protected from damage or discomfort."

Insulated probes are available to electrologists nationwide, and they are one piece of equipment I would insist upon.

Finally, Terri shaved the hair she didn't get to this time so I could be sure I was happy with the shape and told me how many more treatments would be needed.

"When we promise a client a completion date, we are committed to keeping our promise," states Peters emphatically. "The patient, however, must also do her part."

My part consisted of sticking to the agreed-on schedule. And to keep the sessions to a minimum, the only way I was to remove hair was by clipping or shaving.

"At any given time only one-half of your hair is in an

active growth phase—the only time it can be permanently removed," Peters explains. "For the rest we must wait until it is out of the dormant phase. If you pluck or wax, you'll have to wait 13 extra weeks until those hairs have grown above the surface of the skin again." Terri suggested that a week before my next treatment I clip back the unwanted hairs. I did, and by my appointment the hairs in the growth stage were stubbly. These were the ones she removed.

As before, my brows became sensitive and bumpy. Most of the bumps were gone within a half hour, and they were all gone by the time I got home.

The job was complete after six more treatments. At each session, I tried a different technician and had different degrees of discomfort. But the pain was always easily bearable. And there was no regrowth.

Many variables affect how much discomfort you experience. Some people are simply more aware of pain. Some areas of the body are more sensitive, and any area can become more sensitized with continued treatment. These factors you can't help. But you can control your choice of electrologist and the type of equipment used.

"If the discomfort of treatment is closer to pain, or there is regrowth, switch to another electrologist," Peters cautions. "If a bump persists, have it checked by a dermatologist to be sure it's not scarring. Pain, regrowth, and scarring should be things of the past."

I agree. In fact, with the right electrologist, I'd gladly do it all over again.

CHAPTER 34

Don't Get Skinned

By Sadja Greenwood, M.D., M.P.H.

Weigh the risks carefully before using these vitamin-A derivatives.

All drugs have side effects, but two new drugs designed to treat acne and wrinkles, Accutane (isotretinoin) and Retin-A (tretinoin), can be hazardous, especially for women. In the last few years, both drugs, which are related to vitamin A, have become well known and controversial—Accutane because it causes severe birth defects if taken by pregnant women and Retin-A because in addition to smoothing facial wrinkles, it causes uncomfortable side effects.

Accutane

Accutane is the first drug proven effective against severe, cystic acne. It reduces the amount of sebum, the thick waxy material that clogs skin glands and causes this condition. Taken for three to five months, its benefits may remain even after it is discontinued.

Although the drug is effective, its potential side effects include fatigue; visual difficulties; liver damage; muscular aching; elevation of blood fats; dry, peeling skin; and fissures in the corners of the mouth. But most serious are the life-threatening birth defects Accutane produces when taken during the first months of pregnancy—severe heart defects, malformed skulls, lack of ears, and other problems. Although the Food and Drug Administration knew about the birth defect problem before approving the drug—and issued warnings—many pregnant women have unwittingly taken it with disastrous results. New labeling requirements may help: Drawings of babies with

Accutane-related defects and physician instructions for a negative pregnancy test before prescribing the drug.

If you're considering Accutane, be sure you're not pregnant before taking the drug. Start taking Accutane only on the third day of a normal period and use abstinence or two forms of reliable contraception to prevent pregnancy. After discontinuing the drug, don't become pregnant right away. The drug's manufacturers suggest one month after discontinuing; cautious dermatologists suggest at least six months. Do not take the drug if you're nursing.

Retin-A

This topical acne drug has recently received attention for its ability to smooth wrinkles and fade age spots. A small amount applied once a day decreases the formation of waxy skin gland plugs and stimulates the formation of new skin cells and a "rosy glow." When applied daily, Retin-A causes stinging, increased skin warmth, and initial aggravation of acne. Within three to five weeks, the skin usually improves. Users may experience heightened sun sensitivity and need to wear an SPF 15 sun block or discontinue use during summer.

Scientists believe Retin-A's "anti-aging" effect is the result of its ability to stimulate the growth of tiny new blood vessels. Some experts speculate this action may prevent or retard skin cancers; others believe it may stimulate cancer growth. One of Retin-A's biggest problems is that it can cause severe inflammatory problems: irritation, swelling, and scaling of the skin.

Safer Alternatives

While these drugs are effective and certainly have their place in dermatological treatment, there are safer alternatives. Most cases of acne can be helped with topical agents such as benzoyl peroxide (found in over-the-counter preparations such as Clearasil and Oxy 5 and 10). In some cases, antibiotics may be needed. If none of these work, ask your dermatologist about the risks and benefits of using Retin-A, which is effective and doesn't have the severe systemic side effects of Accutane. In women, acne often flares up at ovulation and during menstruation when hormone levels change.

The best approach to skin aging is prevention. While many effects of aging are biologically programmed, skin aging involves a combination of the aging process and accumulated environmental damage, mostly from sunlight. For youthful-looking skin, avoid sunbathing and tanning salons. Wear protective sunblock when you're outside between 10 A.M. and 4 P.M., especially if you're around light reflected off water or snow. Avoid smoking and excess alcohol, which damage the skin. Eat a diet rich in beta-carotene and vitamin C, both found in deeply colored vegetables. If you decide to use Retin-A, use it carefully, under the guidance of a dermatologist familiar with its side effects.

Index